Fortschritte der
Urologie und Nephrologie

Advances in
Urology and Nephrology

543 - 26.Nov.1981 - 1.006

X, 112 Seiten, 45 Abb. u. 43 Tab.

Kunststoff DM 35,-- / 260 g

Gesamtherstellung: Mono-Satzbetrieb

Darmstadt-Arhielgen

Harnsteinsymposien Bonn – Wien

Organisation: W. Vahlensieck, Bonn
G. Gasser, Wien

International workshop held in Tel-Aviv
on December 10-11, 1980

Uric acid lithiasis

Edited by O. Sperling and W. Vahlensieck

With 45 figures and 43 tables

Steinkopff · Darmstadt 1981

CIP-Kurztitelaufnahme der Deutschen Bibliothek

Uric acid lithiasis: [internat. workshop, held in Tel-Aviv on 10th and 11th December 1980]/ ed. by O. Sperling and W. Vahlensieck. – Darmstadt: Steinkopff, 1981.
(Advabces un zrology and nephrology; 16)
(Harnsteinsymposien Bonn–Wien)

ISBN-13: 978-3-7985-0594-0 e-ISBN-13: 978-3-642-85318-0
DOI: 10.1007/978-3-642-85318-0

NE: Sperling, Oded [Hrsg.]; Fortschritte der Urologie und Nephrologie

Softcover reprint of the hardcover 1st edition 1981

Type-Setting and Printing: betz-druck gmbh, D-6100 Darmstadt 12

Preface

Kidney stones is a common and ancient disease. Yet, many questions concerning their etiology, treatment, and prevention are still open. The Harnstein-Symposien Bonn–Wien is an organization designed to bring together scientists from the various fields relevant to urolithiasis: medicine, urology, biochemistry, etc. In the framework of this organization an International Workshop was held in Tel Aviv on December 10 and 11 1980 to discuss the various aspects of uric acid lithiasis.

Uric acid stones have been known to mankind for thousands of years. Urate-containing stones were found in Egyptian mummies and in a three-thousand-year old mummy from Arizona. Evidently, with the constant increase in standard of living, associated with increased amount of purine intake, which we are facing in this century, the frequency of uric acid lithiasis is on the increase. In the second half of this century, significant progress has been made in the knowledge of the mechanisms of uric acid overproduction, as well as in the understanding of the etiology, prevention, and tretament of uric acid stones. As a result, uric acid lithiasis can be prevented and when present it can be treated well. Moreover most uric acid stones can be dissolved in vivo.

This workshop included reviews from some of the leading authorities on the various aspects of uric acid metabolism in man: biochemistry, pathology, renal handling, nutrition, etc., and these reviews and results of new studies are presented here.

We think that the proceedings will enrich our knowledge and stimulate our imagination for new ideas and experiments which will further improve the means of treatment and prevention of uric acid stones.

The workshop was generously supported by the following organizations and all participants would like to express their gratitude to them:
Deutsche Wellcome, Burgwedel
Hoyer, Neuss
Madaus, Cologne
Temmler-Werke, Marburg

We are also grateful to Steinkopff Verlag for publishing the proceedings of the workshop.

The Editors

Contents

List of contributors and participants

Germany

Bach, Dr. D., Urolog. Universitätsklinik Bonn, D-5300 Bonn 1 Venusberg
Bichler, Prof. Dr. K.H., Lehrstuhl u. Abteilung für Urologie der Universität Tübingen, D-7400 Tübingen
Braun, Prof. Dr. J., Urolog. Klinik, Allg. Krankenhaus Untere Sandstr. 32, D-8600 Bamberg
Guttmann, Dr. W., Urology Clinic, Gießen University, D-6300 Gießen, Hinter der Ostanlage 5
Hesse, Dr. rer. nat. A., Urologische Universitätsklinik Bonn, D-5300 Bonn 1 Venusberg
Hicking, Dipl. Biol. W., Urologische Universitätsklinik Bonn, D-5300 Bonn 1 Venusberg
Kahle, Dr. F., Dr. Madaus & Co., Postfach 93 20 01, D-5000 Köln 91
Leskovar, Dr. P., Urologische Klinik und Poliklinik rechts der Isar der Technischen Universität, D-8000 München
Löffler, Dr. W., Medizinische Poliklinik der Universität, Pettenkoferstr. 8a, D-8000 München 2
Lux, Dr. B., Urolog. Klinik, Allg. Krankenhaus Untere Sandstr. 32, D-8600 Bamberg
May, Prof. Dr. P., Urolog. Klinik, Allg. Krankenhaus Untere Sandstr. 32, D-8600 Bamberg
Monreal, A., Dr. Madaus & Co., Postfach 93 20 01, D-5000 Köln 91
Schneeberger, Dr. W., Rehabilitationskrankenhaus Bornheim-Merten, D-5303 Bornheim-Merten
Scholz, Dr. D., Chir. und Urolog. Universitätsklinik Mineralstoffwechsel und Hormonlabor, D-8520 Erlangen
Stockhausen, Dr. G., Deutsche Wellcome GmbH, Postfach 109, D-3006 Burgwedel 1
Strenge, Dipl. oec. troph. A., Urolog. Universitätsklinik Bonn, D-5300 Bonn 1 Venusberg
Vahlensieck, Prof. Dr. W., Urolog. Universitätsklinik Bonn, D-5300 Bonn 1 Venusberg

Switzerland

Roch-Ramel, Prof. Dr. F., Institut de Pharmacologie Universite de Lausanne, Lausanne

Sweden

Backman, Dr. U., Department of Internal Medicine, University Hospital, S-750 14 Uppsala
Fellström, Dr. B., Department of Internal Medicine, University Hospital S0750 14 Uppsala

USA

Kelley, Prof. Dr. W.N., University of Michigan, Medical School, Dep. Internal Medicine, Ann. Arbor, Mi 48109
Wyngaarden, Prof. Dr. J.B., Duke University Medical Center, Durham, N.C. 27710

Austria

Deetjen, Prof. Dr. P., Institut f. Physiologie der Universität Innsbruck, A-6010 Innsbruck
Joost, Dr. J., Urolog. Universitätsklinik Innsbruck, A-6010 Innsbruck

U.K.

Simmonds, Dr. H.A., Guy's Hospital Medical School, Purine laboratory, London Bridge, London SE, 9RT

Israel

De Vries, Prof. Dr. A., 10 Melchet St. Tel-Aviv
Halabe, Dr. A., Beilinson Medical Center Metabolic Unit, Petah-Tikva
Rosenfeld, Prof. Dr. J., Beilinson Medical Center, Dept. of Medicine C and Nephrology, Petah-Tikva
Samuel, Dr. R., Beilinson Medical Center, Metabolic Unit, Petah-Tikva
Servadio, Prof. Dr. C., Beilinson Medical Center, Dept. of Urol. Petah-Tikva
Sperling, Prof. Dr. O., Beilinson Medical Center, Dept. Clinical Biochemistry, Petah-Tikva

Fortschritte der Urol. und Nephrol. **16**, 1–4 (1981)
Steinkopff Verlag Darmstadt

Hyperuricemia-Epidemiology 1980

G. Stockhausen

Deutsche Wellcome, Burgwedel

Introduction

In the last thirty years, data which have been published on the level of serum uric acid in man have varied considerably. The main reason for this is a considerable increase in the uric acid values. Furthermore, different laboratory methods (mostly improved laboratory techniques), the selection of the treatment groups, the different definition of the critical value, which is often mistaken for the middle or average value, and last but not least the different conditions for blood taking have all been responsible for these variable data.

Definition

Critical for the definition of hyperuricemia is always the solubility of uric acid or its salts in serum; this is a biochemical value, which is commonly calculated as 6.4 mg% (380 μmol/liter) and is the same for both males and females. Uric acid values exceeding this pathological limit of 6.4 mg% in serum are therefore critical, as uric acid is then able to crystallize, especially in the bradytropnic tissue. Furthermore this mechanism is supported by a move of the pH value to the acid range induced by the uric acid itself.

History

In 1848 Garrod recognized hyperuricemia as the cause of gout, which is the pathological final state of a long – usually more than 10 years – existing hyperuricemia. The level of uric acid in serum varies individually between 3 and 6 mg%. Today the average in males is about 5.5 mg% and in young females about 4.4 mg% with slight deviations due to the daily rhythm. 400–600 mg uric acid are excreted daily into the urine and 20% are catabolized by bacteria in the gut. A hyperuricosuria is considered to be present when the uric acid level is more than 600 mg in the 24-hour urine. This is an essential parameter for the growth of uric acid and uric acid combination stones.
Here is a short but most fascinating look at the history of evolution: With the stepwise loss of the enzyme uricase the quantity of uric acid increases along with further development. Very low uric acid quantities are found in lower mammals, for example porpoises (other values are 0.2 mg% in lemurs, 1.0 mg% in monkeys, and 2 mg% in anthropoids).
Hyperuricemia depends on: genetic factors, age, diet, alcohol, psychological and physical overload, stress, diseases (for example, polycythemia, ketose), and drugs (for example, thiacides).

Epidemiology

Long years of starvation and privation in Europe have been overcompensated with excessive "good eating and drinking." Hyperuricemia has increased in adults as follows: from 0.05 to 0.1% (gout 0.01%) in 1950, to 10% in 1960, and to 20% in 1970. With varying values in males and females, volunteers (e.g. blood donors) and patients in practices and hospitals.

Zöllner in Munich, carried out an interesting comparative trial in 999 blood donors. He found a uric-acid-plasma-level above 6.5 mg% in 8% of 1961 males, 4% of 1961 females (total = 12%), 19.2% of 1971 males, and 4.3% of 1971 females (total = 23.5%).

To check on the present-day occurrence of hyperuricemia in adults, uric acid values were investigated for 6 months in two general practices, in a collective laboratory for practitioners, in a medical laboratory (as well as from data from other practitioners and small private hospitals), two clinics, and in blood donors.

All analyses were carried out enzymatically under control. The following are simplified data:

1. Two *general practices:*

	Practice 1	Practice 2
Approximate number of patients per month	1000	1200
Approximate number of uric acid examinations per month	100	40
Percentages of patients with hyperuricemia	23%	30%

Practice 1 Percentages of patients with uric acid levels above	6.5 mg% = 23.2%	above 8 mg% = 6.7%	above 9 mg% = 2.1%
Practice 2 Percentages of patients with uric acid levels above	6.5 mg% = 30.1%	above 8 mg% = 9.2%	above 9 mg% = 3.9%
Average	= 26.6%	= 7.9%	= 3.0%

These three groups of hyperuricemia not only have historical, statistical, and academic value for the doctor but are also of practial value. In the sense of modern preventive medicine all hyperuricemic patients firstly require specified examinations for other metabolic disorders and secondly corresponding advice and treatment.

2. Two *laboratories* (collective and medical):

	Laboratory 1	Laboratory 2
Approximate number of uric acid examinations per month	1000	600
Percentages of patients with hyperuricemia	24.1%	21.1%

Laboratory 1 Percentages of patients with uric acid levels above	6.5 mg% = 24.1%	above 8 mg% = 9.9%	above 9 mg% = 4.5%
Laboratory 2 Percentages of patients with uric acid levels above	6.5 mg% = 21.1%	above 8 mg% = 7.4%	above 9 mg% = 3.7%
Average	= 22.6%	= 8.9%	= 4.1%

3. In the two *clinics,* about 2200 uric acid investigations per month were carried out in clinic 1 and 2500 in clinic 2 with the help of MSA (in each patient only the first measurement was taken into consideration).

	Clinic 1	Clinic 2
Percentages of patients with hyperuricemia	29.3%	21.1%

Clinic 1			
Percentages of patients with uric acid levels above	6.8 mg% = 29.3%	above 8 mg% = 12.7%	above 9 mg% = 5.7%
Percentages of patients with uric acid levels above	6.8 mg% = 21.1%	above 8 mg% = 7.4%	above 9 mg% = 3.7%
Average	= 25.2%	= 10.1%	= 4.7%

In a group of 8625 *blood donors* the following uric acid values were measured in 6223 males: 6.8 mg% in 21.5%, 8 mg% in 6.0%, and 9 mg% in 1.7%. The various age groups of those males showed a slight but continuous increase from 20.1% to 23.6%. In females there was a considerable increase of hyperuricemia from 2.1% to 6.7% starting at the age of 50.

Risk Factors

The frequent correlation with other diseases makes hyperuricemia an important risk factor. Correlations are as follows:

1. hypertension = 55%
2. overweight (adipositas) = 50%
3. hepatopathy = 40%
4. nephropathy = 35%
5. vascular diseases = 35%
6. hyperlipemia = 25%
7. diabetes = 8% (subclinical = 15%)
8. nephrolithiasis = 8%

Our data 1980 are given in Table 1.

Table 1: Risk factors

	Practice 1	Practice 2	Laboratory 1	Laboratory 2	Hospital 1	Hospital 2
Serum uric acid over 6.5 mg%	30%	22%	24%	18%	29%	21%
Cholesterol over 250 mg%	39%	31%	32%	27%	30%	25%
Triglyceride over 180 mg%	51%	44%	45%	35%	33%	29%
Creatinine over 1.4 mg%	–	–	43%	39%	50%	44%

In general practice a significant increase of cholesterol of 39% and of triglyceride of 51% was found. Creatinine values were also increased in laboratory and clinic. Hyperuricemia is a risk with regard to its level and a great risk especially in connection with other metabolic pathological parameters. These patients have to be controlled for

a long time to prevent kidney damage, kidney stones, and vascular diseases occurring, particularly as nowadays a successful therapy is available.

Summary

The concentration of uric acid in serum is the complex result of several endogenous and exogenous factors. For biochemical reasons, a hyperuricemia is said to occur if the uric acid level in serum exceeds 6.5 mg% (387 μmol/liter). It was difficult previously to interpret epidemiological average values because of the different laboratory methods and different limiting values of 6.0 to 8.0 mg% used by different research groups. However, all investigations have shown an enormous increase of hyperuricemia in Europe in recent decades from 0.1% in adults in 1950 to nearly 10% in 1960 and 20% in 1970. Therefore we explored the serum uric acid levels for a period of 6 months in 1980 in 2 general practices, in 2 laboratories, in 2 hospitals, and in blood donors. In two general practices hyperuricemia (⩾ 6.5 mg%) was found in 21.1% of all patients, in the hospitals in 25.2% of all patients; in male blood donors in 21.5% and in female blood donors in 3.3%. These results show that in the last decade the trend toward a further increase in uric acid has dimished. Furthermore the coincidence of hyperuricemia and other pathological laboratory parameters has been examined. A significant frequency was found if there was an increase in creatinine and triglycerides. A partial increase has also been stated with SGOT and cholesterol. Hyperuricemia is not a disease but a pathological condition, the causes of which have to be clarified.

Author's address:

Dr. Georg Stockhausen
Deutsche Wellcome GmbH
3006 Burgwedel 1
Germany

Fortschritte der Urol. und Nephrol. **16**, 5–7 (1981)
Steinkopff Verlag Darmstadt

Control of Purine Biosynthesis

James B. Wyngaarden

Duke University Medical Center, Durham, N. C., U.S.A.

The feedback inhibition of the first specific enzyme of purine biosynthesis, amidophosphoribosyltransferase, by the purine ribonucleotides AMP and GMP was described in a partially purified enzyme system over 20 years ago(1). The molecular basis for this inhibition, namely the aggregation of active subunits to an enzymatically inactive larger form in the presence of purine ribonucleotides, was described with the amidophosphoribosyltransferase obtained from human placenta seven years ago(2). Phosphoribosylpyrophosphate (PRPP) activates the mammalian enzyme by causing disaggregation of the inhibited large form to the catalytically active small form.

The relative importance of feedback inhibition and substrate activation of amidophosphoribosyltransferase in the control of purine biosynthesis de novo has been difficult to sort out, and indeed could vary in different tissues or even in the same tissue at different times and under different circumstances.

There has also been considerable interest in the enzyme catalyzing the immediately preceding step, namely phosphoribosylpyrophosphate synthetase, an enzyme also subject to complex regulation including activation by inorganic phosphate and inhibition by purine ribonucleotides. In some studies in tissue culture, e.g., those of Sperling and colleagues in skin fibroblasts(3) and in epithelial-like rat liver cells(4), the activation of this enzyme and the rate of PRPP synthesis appeared to be the limiting and controlling factors for purine ribonucleotide synthesis, whereas in other studies, such as those of Hershfield and Seegmiller(5) in the WI-L2 line of diploid human lymphoblasts (5) and of Allsop and Watts in unstimulated and stimulated human lymphocytes (6), PRPP did not appear to play a central role and end-product feedback regulatory effects were thought to be more important for coordination of purine nucleotide synthesis.

Because of the varied results and opinions on the relative roles of PRPP and purine ribonucleotides in the control of purine biosynthesis, Holmes and his group at Duke University decided to study this problem in the liver of an intact animal given fructose to stimulate purine production. It is well known that intravenous fructose administration results in intracellular purine ribonucleotide breakdown and hyperuricemia with a subsequent increase in purine biosynthesis de novo (7, 8, 9). Holmes reasoned that if these effects could be reproduced in the mouse, and appropriate measurements made, further information on regulation of the early steps of purine biosynthesis might be obtained. Accordingly, mice were injected intravenously with fructose or glucose, and after variable intervals of time, the animals were anesthetized with ether, and their livers freeze clamped in liquid nitrogen in vivo. The frozen livers were used for determination of purine ribonucleotides by high-pressure liquid chromatography, of PRPP content by enzymatic assay, and of amidophosphoribosyltransferase conformation by gel filtration.

Preliminary studies showed that the incorporation of [^{14}C]-glycine into hepatic purines was five times greater in the mice receiving fructose than in those given glucose; thus there was good evidence that purine biosynthesis de novo had been greatly stimulated following fructose infusion relative to that following glucose infusion.

A surprising initial finding was that the amidophosphoribosyltransferase was largely in the *inactive* form in resting mouse liver. About 93 to 95 percent of the enzyme was regularly found to be in the large or catalytically inactive form prior to glucose or fructose infusion. By thirty minutes after fructose infusion the amidophosphoribosyltransferase had undergone a marked change in conformation, and over 30 percent was now in the small or enzymatically active form. Glucose infusion resulted in no change in conformation of the enzyme. So now Holmes had an intact mammalian system in which fructose but not glucose caused accelerated purine biosynthesis de novo, as assessed by glycine incorporation into hepatic purines, that appeared to be correlated with a marked shift of form of the first enzyme of the pathway from an inactive to an active state. Such a shift of form could theoretically be brought about by a decrease in purine ribonucleotide concentration or an increase in PRPP concentration or by some combination of these two effects.

The total purine nucleotide constant of mouse liver fell within three minutes of fructose infusion, and remained at the reduced level for at least 30 minutes. The total nucleotide content fell after glucose infusion also, although somewhat less than after fructose. However, ADP content did not fall after glucose, whereas it fell significantly after fructose, and when the nucleotide changes were expressed in terms of "inhibitory potential" for amidophosphoribosyltransferase, that is, specifically in terms of those ribonucleotides that inhibit the enzymes such as AMP and GMP, this inhibitory potential fell only following fructose infusion. The fall was statistically significant at 30 minutes.

Cellular PRPP concentrations also changed following fructose infusion, approximately doubling in 30 minutes. They did not change significantly following glucose infusion. Thus fructose infusion lowered intracellular AMP, GMP, and ADP concentrations; raised intracellular PRPP concentrations; and markedly increased purine biosynthesis de novo. Holmes' concept of how this comes about is as follows: The rapid phosphorylation of fructose lowers intracellular levels of ATP. This is restored from ADP by nucleoside diphosphokinase, with loss of considerable AMP from the cell through action of 5' nucleotidases. The reduction in ADP and other nucleotides releases PRPP synthetase from inhibition resulting in increased synthesis of PRPP. The reduction in AMP and the increase in PRPP together activate amidophosphoribosyltransferase by shifting its conformation from the large inactive to the small catalytically active form, leading to increased synthesis of phosphoribosylamine and of purine ribonucleotides. Thus PRPP synthetase and amidophosphoribosyltransferase may be coordinately regulated through sequential and complex allosteric effects. At least in this system, control does not seem to be invested in PRPP concentrations alone, nor in ribonucleotide concentrations alone, nor in either enzyme alone.

Previous attempts to address this problem have shown no increase in specific activity of PRPP synthetase or amidophosphoribosyltransferase under conditions of stimulation of purine production (6). But in these studies enzyme assays were conducted under activating conditions in the assay cuvette. The present study (10) demonstrates that marked changes of enzyme activity can be brought about in vivo by allosteric effects that would not be detected by routine assays and that require conditions which allow recognition of the physical and catalytic state of the enzyme in the tissue at the moment of analysis. We believe that this study has made a further contribution to the interesting topic of control of purine biosynthesis, and thereby to the problem of uric acid lithiasis.

References

1. Wyngaarden, J.B. and Ashton, D.M.: J. Biol. Chem. **234:** 1492, 1959.
2. Holmes, E.W., Wyngaarden, J.B. and Kelley, W.N.: J. Biol. Chem. **248:** 6035, 1973.
3. Zoref-Shani, E. and Sperling, O.: Biochim Biophys Acta **607:** 503, 1980.
4. Bashkin, P. and Sperling, O.: Biochim Biophys Acta **538:** 505, 1978.
5. Hershfield, M.S. and Seegmiller, J.E.: J. Biol. Chem. **252:** 6002, 1977.
6. Allsop, J. and Watts, R.W.E.: M. Molec. Med. **3:** 105, 1978.
7. Fox, I.H. and Kelley, W.N.: Metabolism **21:** 713, 1972.
8. Bode, J.C., Zelder, O., Rumpelt, H.J.: Eur. J. Clin. Invest. **3:** 436, 1973.
9. Schwarzmeier, J.D., Marktl, W., Moserk and Luif, A.: Res. Exp. Med. **162:** 341, 1974.
10. Itakura, M., Sabina, R.L., Heald, P.W., Holmes, E.W.: **67:** 994, 1981. J. Clin. Invest., 1980.

Author's address:

Prof. Dr. *James B. Wyngaarden*
Duke University Medical Center
Durham, N.C. 27710
USA

Fortschritte der Urol. und Nephrol. **16**, 8–18 (1981)
Steinkopff Verlag Darmstadt

Nutrition and Uric Acid Metabolism: Plasma Level, Turnover Excretion

W. Löffler, W. Gröbner, and N. Zöllner

Medizinische Poliklinik der Universität München, West Germany

In order to evaluate the influence of nutrition on uric acid formation and eventual excretion, adequate methods must be used. They may be based on two different principles, those of metabolic balance on the one hand and isotope incorporation and subsequent dilution on the other.

Balance experiments produce results that can be interpreted only if (or when) a steady state is obtained, because only then does the input from any source equal output. The example of the fountain serves well. As long as the level in the trough rises or falls, the inflow cannot easily be ascertained from the coutflow. In uric acid metabolism inflow is from exogenous and endogenous sources, outflow is throught the kidneys and the gastrointestinal tract only because metabolic degradation is considered minimal or absent. For steady-state conditions it is irrelevant whether there is one pool or a group of pools (Fig. 1).

In experiments, a steady state appears to be obtained if all parameters measurable become constant. With respect to uric acid excretion or uric acid level in plasma, equilibrium is reached after 7 days. Therefore, results from balance experiments can only be used such an interval. Reports which do not consider this should be disregarded.

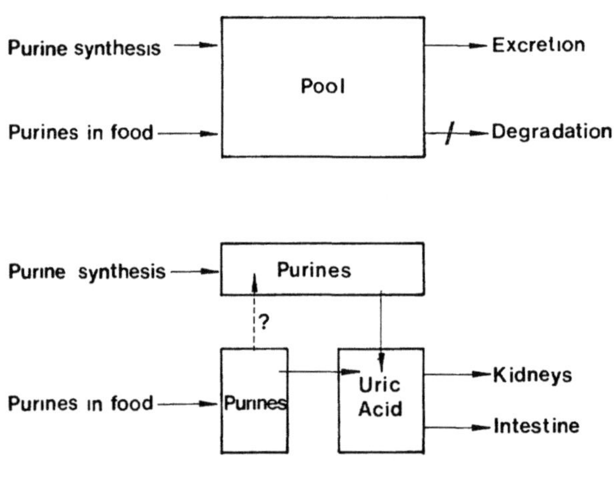

Fig. 1: Synthesis of purines and purines in food both contribute to the purine and uric acid pool(s), respectively. Nothing is known about interrelations between the purines of different origin. Excretion of the end-product uric acid occurs via the kidneys and the intestinal tract, while no degradation takes place in vivo.

Reservations concerning the interpretation of isotope experiments have been clearly discussed previously (Bishop et al., 1951; Zöllner, 1960).

1. Endogenous uric acid production

We recently summarized (Table 1) the data of 36 normal subjects who had eaten a purine-free, isoenergetic liquid formula diet for at least 7 days. It is obvious from these data, that endogenous uric acid production is considerably lower than was generally assumed in the recent past. And this of course also means that serum uric acid levels can be lowered to a great degree by dietary means in patients who do not overproduce uric acid endogenously. Excretion values found by Burian and Schur (1900) are within the range of studies performed during low-purine diets.

Table 1: Serum and urinary uric acid values in normal subjects during their personal diet and after 7 days of ingestion of an isoenergetic, purine-free liquid formula diet.

	Females (n = 11) conventional diet	formula diet	Males (n = 25) conventional diet	formula diet
Serum uric acid (mg/100 ml)	4.22 ± 0.50	3.28 ± 0.68	5.42 ± 0.84	4.03 ± 0.74
Urinary uric acid (mg/day)	453 ± 99	252 ± 67	548 ± 197	321 ± 87

In Fig. 2 the decrease in renal excretion after commencing the purine-free diet is shown. When these experimental data were corrected for body weight, there was a tendency of the females to excrete more endogenous uric acid renally than the male subjects (not significant), while per body surface no difference could be seen between the sexes. However, the plasma levels in females were significantly lower, demonstrating an increased endogenous uric acid clearance in young women. A geater uric acid clearance in women has previously been noted (Wolfson et al., 1949; Scott and Pollard, 1970), but never on a purine-free diet.

There are only a few uric acid data of gout patients on a low-purine diet or an a purine-free diet. Seegmiller et al. (1961) found that the percentage reduction of serum uric acid on a low-purine diet was the same in gouty and normal subjects, which means that in absolute figures the reduction is greater in gout than in normal subjects. In this century the experiences of the two World Wars clearly showed that gout can be prevented by dietary means. We therefore conclude that on an appropriate diet not only normal but also gouty subjects will have normal serum uric acid levels, those of gouty patients being slightly higher (Fig. 3).

2. Dietary purines and uric acid metabolism

Soon after the chemical structure of uric acid had been established in 1898 (Fischer, 1907), Burian and Schur (1900, 1901, 1903) were able to show that uric acid in humans was derived from endogenous production as well as from dietary sources.

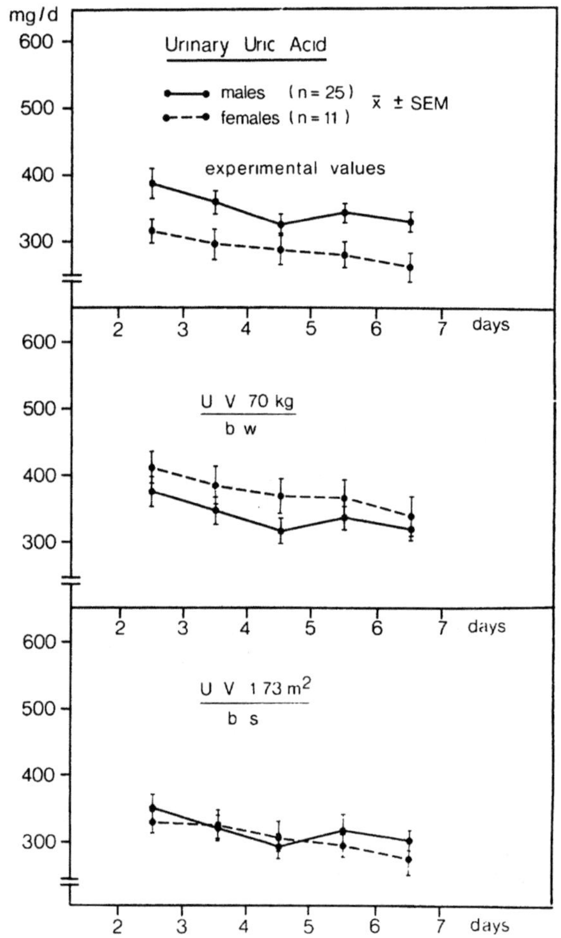

Fig. 2: Decrease of renal uric acid excretion during an isoenergetic, purine-free liquid formula diet. There is a significant difference between males and females in experimental values. This is no longer present when the data are corrected for body surface.

2.1 Influence on serum and urinary uric acid levels

Nugent and Tyler (1959) were the first to evaluate the influence of defined dietary purines on uric acid metabolism after specific methods for uric acid estimations had become available. They added different doses of ribonucleic acid (RNA) to a low-purine diet and found an increase in serum and urinary uric acid with increasing amounts of RNA. This soon became a standard method in studies of uric acid metabolism. A dose of 4 g RNA has been used by various authors to produce mild hyperuricemia in normal subjects (Table 2).

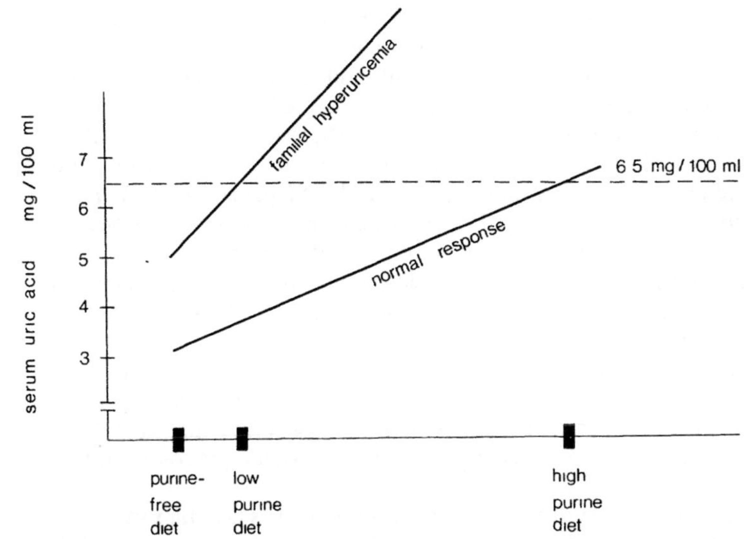

Fig. 3: The different response of serum uric acid levels to dietary purines in familial hyperuricemia compared with normal subjects.

Table 2: Serum uric acid concentrations during the administration of a basal diet (low-purine diet) and during addition of 4 g ribonucleic acid per day in normal subjects.

Reference		Serum uric acid (mg/100 ml) low-purine diet	4 g RNA/day
Seegmiller et al.,	1962	4.6	8.19
Nugent et al.,	1964	4.88	7.4
Waslien et al.,	1968	4.9	7.68
Waslien et al.,	1970	5.4	8.7
Griebsch and Zöllner,	1970	4.5	7.44

There was a different response to RNA in gouty patients compared with normals. Characteristically patients with familial hyperuricemia and gout have higher serum uric acid levels at the same renal excretion, and a lower renal excretion at the same serum level. Accordingly, with RNA added to the diet, serum uric acid levels increased more in gouty patients than in normals (Nugent et al., 1964; Griebsch and Zöllner, 1970).

After the effect of dietary RNA had been well established, Zöllner and his co-workers (Griebsch and Zöllner, 1971; Zöllner et al., 1972) investigated the influence of different dietary purine compounds on uric acid metabolism. It was found that the size of the response depended on the source of the purines. For example the increase in serum and urine uric acid was less with DNA than that produced by RNA, while it was greater with nucleotides. When single cell protein was added to a standard diet, the effect was greater than that of DNA, but less than that of RNA, which was to be expected from

the content of DNA and RNA of this kind of food. There was a linear increase of uric acid with increasing purine doses in both serum and urine.
The response of serum and urine uric acid to different kinds of dietary purines was explained by the hypothesis that RNA and DNA have to be degraded to their nucleotides (and possibly nucleosides) prior to absorption, and that different absorption might be due to a different velocity of degradation. This results in a renal excretion of the purines administered orally of about 25 percent in the case of DNA, 50 percent with RNA, and 80 percent with nucleotides (Zöllner et al., 1972). The conclusion drawn from these results was that only nucleotides are absorbed from the gut completely.
We have also administered different purine nucleosides to healthy volunteers. Preliminary data show that the changes in serum and urine uric acid levels are comparable to those achieved by administration of purine nucleotides.
It is well known that on a vegetarian diet gout is rare compared with a diet rich in meat. However, isoenergetic amounts of meat and vegetables contain roughly the same amounts of RNA purine nitrogen (Zöllner and Griebsch, 1973). It was assumed that the relatively high content of ATP degradation products in meat might contribute predominantly to hyperuricemia.
As hypoxanthine is an end product of purine metabolism in tissues lacking xanthine oxidase, we investigated the concentration of hypoxanthine in meat, and compared this with the effects seen after oral administration of hypoxanthine (Spann et al., 1980). The hypoxanthine content of pork increased with time of storage and with temperature. The nutrition experiment showed that the content of 200 g of barely edible pork resulted in an increase in serum uric acid of only 0.15 mg/100 ml. This was less than the increase produced by RNA.
When other purine bases were investigated, there was a different effect on uric acid metabolism with each of the compounds. In one healthy subject there was only a very small increase in serum and urinary uric acid during the administration of guanine (Gröbner et al., unpublished results), whereas guanine hydrochloride seems to be better absorbed (Simmonds et al., 1973). Adenine seems to be absorbed very well from the gut in both animal (Potter et al., 1980) and man (Gröbner et al., unpublished), but is metabolized differently leading to a greater percentage of hypoxanthine in the total oxipurine excretion.
To summarize the data on endogenous uric acid production and on purine supplementation experiments, it would appear that on an average diet about half the urinary uric acid and one-third of the plasma uric acid is derived from dietary purine compounds in normal man. These contribute to the increase in serum uric acid and renal excretion of uric acid according to the velocity of their enzymatic hydrolysis within the intestine and also according to their solubility and degree of absorption.

2.2. Turnover of endogenous and exogenous uric acid

On a diet free of purines, renal uric acid clearance is lower than on a conventional diet. The administration of purines leads to an increase of uric acid clearance. From the increased renal uric acid clearance it can be concluded that the turnover rate of the uric acid pool is increased, provided the intestinal uric acid clearance remains constant or is increased as well.

The turnover rate as measured by the isotope dilution method of Benedict and coworkers (1949) estimates the fraction of the uric acid pool which is replaced by newly synthetized uric acid per day. This means that it is a measure of total body uric acid clearance.

Bowering et al. (1969) studied two normal subjects on a low-purine diet as well as on an oral load of 4 g RNA by the isotope dilution technique. The two subjects were of the same age and body weight. However, there was a considerable difference in response to RNA as far as turnover rate was concerned (Table 3). In one subject the change in turnover rate was near the range of error for the method, while in the second there was an increase of about 40 percent.

Table 3: Changes in uric acid pool size and turnover rate in normal subjects induced by oral purine administration.

	Pool size (mg)		Turnover rate (pools/day)	
Ref. (Dietary purine source)	control	purine supplementation	control	purine supplementation
Bowering et al., 1969 (RNA)	1060 767	2127 1580	0.61 0.65	0.66 0.92
Löffler et al., 1980a (AMP, GMP)	569 684 562	763 1592 1325	0.82 0.66 0.63	1.21 0.81 0.85

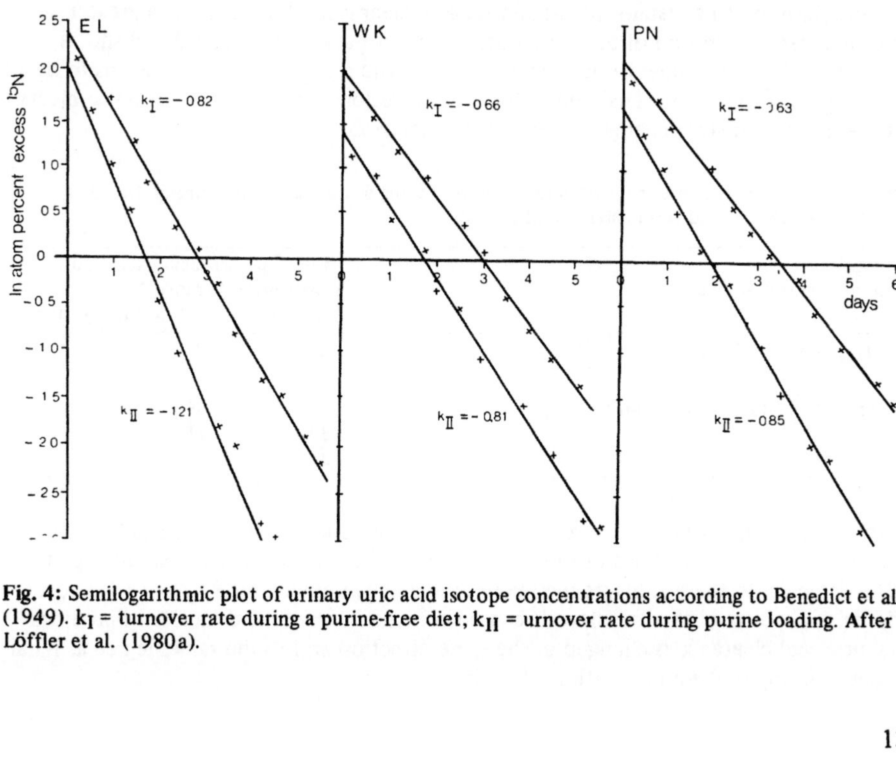

Fig. 4: Semilogarithmic plot of urinary uric acid isotope concentrations according to Benedict et al. (1949). k_I = turnover rate during a purine-free diet; k_{II} = urnover rate during purine loading. After Löffler et al. (1980a).

We recently investigated the effect of oral purines on uric acid pool size and turnover rate in three normal subjects (Löffler et al., 1980a). The diet was an isoenergetic liquid formula diet free of purines and the purine supplement was 1 g AMP plus 1 g GMP per 70 kg body weight, which corresponds to about 4 g RNA as used by Bowering et al. (1969). Results are shown in Table 3 and in Fig. 4. It is obvious that in normal subjects dietary purines lead to an increase in turnover rate of uric acid pool.

In familial gout and hyperuricemia renal uric acid clearance is diminished compared with normals. It can be concluded from this that the turnover rate of the miscible uric acid pool is also diminished in gout. Summarizing the literature on uric acid turnover studies, there was a mean turnover rate of 0.46 (± 0.11) pools/day in gout and hyperuricemia (n = 33), while in normal subjects (n = 38) it was 0.60 (± 0.14) pools/day ($p < 0.001$). However, data reported on renal function of the subjects were insufficient in some of these publications to exclude secondary renal disease. The difference might therefore be due, at least in part, to renal insufficiency in patients with gout.

Studies cited above have shown that renal uric acid clearance is enhanced to a lesser degree in gout than in normal humans when RNA is added to the diet. It can be concluded from this that, compared with controls, the turnover rate of the uric acid pool in familial gout is also increased less on dietary purine supplementation.

2.3. Uric acid excretion during oral purine administration

In this part we would like to focus on changes in the percentage of renal and extrarenal uric acid excretion.

As mentioned before renal uric acid clearance is enhanced during oral purine administration. Assuming a constant intestinal uric acid clearance, this results in a greater percentage of renal excretion of uric acid during dietary purine loading. Table 4 shows percentage excretion values derived from isotopic uric acid studies. There seems to be a wide range of variation in renal and extrarenal excretion of uric acid in normal subjects, but there is no constant change in percentage excretion.

Table 4: Estimation of extrarenal uric acid excretion during a low-purine or, a purine-free diet, and during additional oral administration of purines.

Reference (Purine supplement)	Intestinal uric acid excretion (percent of turnover) control	oral purine loading
Bowering et al., 1969 (RNA)	22	25
	54	25
Löffler et al., 1980a (AMP + GMP)	49	36
	39	41
	21	38

To study extrarenal uric acid excretion directly, we gave high doses of antibiotics to three normal subjects during a purine-free diet as well as during an oral load of 4 g of RNA (Table 5). In these subjects the maximum change induced by RNA was 2 percent (Löffler et al., unpublished results). It can be concluded from the data cited that extrarenal uric acid clearance is changed in the same direction and to the same degree as renal clearance during oral administration of purines.

Table 5: Uric acid excretion in urine and feces in normal subjects during intestinal bacteriostasis.

		Uric acid excretion purine-free diet		4 g RNA/day	
Subject		mg/day	percent	mg/day	percent
1	Urine	262	59	680	57
	Feces	186	41	524	43
2	Urine	291	53	784	55
	Feces	255	47	631	45
3	Urine	321	51	526	52
	Feces	313	49	478	48

Antibiotics were administered in 4 daily doses. Daily dosage: Paromomycine, 4.0 g; Ampicilline, 4.0 g; Colistin, 2 mg/kg; Metronidazole, 4.0 g; Nystatine, 3 000 000 I. U. While with a normal intestinal flora uric acid is only inconstantly found in feces, nearly 50 percent of the total excretion of uric acid was found in feces under this regimen.

3. Dietary protein supplementation and uric acid metabolism

3.1. Influence on serum level and renal excretion

Studies at the beginning of this century showed that there was an increase in renal uric acid excretion with increasing amounts of protein in the diet (Taylor and Rose, 1914; Leopold et al., 1925). However, there were controversial results as fas as serum levels were concerned.

Bien et al. (1953) studied one normal subject, and found an increase in renal uric acid excretion of 62 mg/day by nearly doubling the protein content of the diet. At the same time there was an increase in incorporation of ^{15}N-glycine into uric acid, which was attributed to an increased endogenous uric acid synthesis.

If there is an increased uric acid synthesis as well as an additional enhancement of renal excretion, one might expect constant serum levels of uric acid while excretion increases. In agreement with this hypothesis, there were publications which showed a considerable increase in renal excretion of uric acid and at the same time only slight or no variations in serum levels (Bowering et al., 1969).

These authors had used as a control a low-purine diet composed mainly of conventional food and compared it with rather unphysiological diets such as a protein-free and a high-protein diet containing 68 energy percent protein.

Later Matzkies and Berg (1977) administered amino acids intravenously and demonstrated a uricosuric effect of these substances. There was also an increased renal uric acid clearance during oral administration of amino acids and protein, which could have been due to a uricosuric action of amino acids (Yü et al., 1970) and/or an increased glomerular filtration rate (O'Connor and Summerill, 1976).

We therefore reinvestigated this question using a purine-free liquid formula diet containing 12, 24, and 36 energy percent protein (Löffler et al., 1980b). The results of this study are shown in Table 6. It is obvious that not only renal excretion of uric acid increased, but also serum levels decreased under these conditions. We conclude from these results that formula diets give more consistent results in experimental studies than low-purine diets of conventional food.

Table 6: Serum and urinary uric acid values of five healthy subjects during different protein contents of an isoenergetic, purine-free formula diet. The protein content was increased at the expense of fat and carbohydrates in equal amounts of energy. After Löffler et al. (1980b).

	Dietary protein (energy percent) 12	24	36
Serum uric acid (mg/100 ml)	3.72 ± 0.55	2.84 ± 0.60	2.51 ± 0.44
Urinary uric acid (mg/day)	287 ± 48	356 ± 73	386 ± 84

3.2. Uric acid turnover during dietary protein supplementation

We have seen that there is a rise in turnover rate of the uric acid pool when purines are administered orally. In the case of proteins there is an increase in renal excretion as well as a decrease in serum levels. This results in a great enhancement of renal clearance with relatively small changes in protein intake.

It can be concluded from this that the turnover rate of uric acid pool increases more with proteins than with purines added to the diet. This was shown by Bowering et al. (1969), who compared the effects of RNA with those of protein supplementation in normal subjects. When changing from a 90 g protein diet to a diet containing 408 g protein, the pool size was unchanged (what could be expected from the constant serum level), while the turnover rate was doubled (Table 7). When 4 g of RNA were added to the 90 g protein diet, the pool size was nearly doubled, while the turnover rate was unchanged in one subject and rose by 40 percent in the second (see Table 3).

Table 7: Turnover rate of uric acid pool in three normal males during a low-purine, low-protein diet, and during a high-protein diet. After Bowering et al. (1969).

	Turnover rate of uric acid pool (pools/day)	
Subject	control	high-protein diet
3	0.61	1.14
5	0.52	1.01
6	0.65	1.35

3.3. Renal and extrarenal uric acid excretion during dietary protein supplementation

Assuming a constant uric acid production, every uricosuric drug as well as all other measures leading to an increased renal clearance of uric acid alone while the intestinal clearance remains constant will result in a greater proportion of uric acid being excreted renally.

This change was clearly demonstrated in the three normal subjects studied by Bowering et al. (1969). Table 8 compares the effect of protein supplementation with that of uri-

Table 8: Changes in the percentage of renal uric acid excretion during administration of uricosuric durgs and during a high-protein diet.

	Renal excretion of uric acid (percent of turnover)	
	control	uricosuric action
Bishop et al., 1951 b	71.5	89.6
(Probenecide)	98.9[1]	not reported[1]
Wyngaarden, 1955	82	93
(Phenylbutazone)	80	93
Bowering et al., 1969	46	88
	56	78
(dietary proteins[2])	78	86

[1] Gouty subject. All others were normal controls.

[2] Besides uricosuric action there is possibly an additional mechanism contributing to this change.

cosuric drugs. As far as the change in percentage excretion is concerned, no difference between dietary protein and uricosuric drugs can be derived from these results. We therefore conclude that the absence of changes in serum levels during dietary protein supplementation in earlier investigations might have been due to a concomitant increase of purine intake, as these diets were composed of conventional food. At present, a small increase in endogenous uric acid production during dietary protein supplementation cannot be excluded. However, the influence of amino acids on renal uric acid excretion as shown by Yü et al. (1970) and Matzkies and Berg (1977) sufficiently explains the data presently available.

References

1. Benedict, J. D., Forsham, P. H., Stetten, D.: The metabolism of uric acid in the normal and gouty human studied with the aid of isotopic uric acid. J. Biol. Chem. **181:** 183 (1949).
2. Bien, E. J., Yü, T. F., Benedict, J. D., Gutman, A. E., Stetten, D.: The relation of dietary nitrogen consumption to the rate of uric acid synthesis in normal and gouty man. J. Clin. Invest. **32:** 778 (1953).
3. Bishop, Ch., Garner, W., Talbott, J. H.: Pool size, turn-over rate, and rapidity of equilibration of injected isotopic uric acid in normal and pathological subjects. J. Clin. Invest. **30:** 879 (1951 a).
4. Bishop, Ch., Rand, R., Talbott, J. H.: The effect of Benemid on uric acid metabolism in one normal and one gonty subject. J. Clin. Invest. **30:** 889 (1951 b)
5. Bowering, J., Calloway, D. H., Margen, S., Kaufmann, N. A.: Dietary protein level and uric acid metabolism in normal man. J. Nutr. **100:** 249 (1969).
6. Burian, R., Schur, H.: Über die Harnpurinausscheidung des Menschen. Pflugers Archiv **80:** 241 (1900).
7. Burian, R., Schur, H.: Über die Stellung der Purinkörper im menschlichen Stoffwechsel. Pflugers Archiv **87:** 239 (1901).
8. Burian, R., Schur, H.: Das quantitative Verhalten der menschlichen Harnpurin-Ausscheidung. Pflügers Archiv **94:** 273 (1903).
9. Fischer, E.: Untersuchungen in der Puringruppe. Springer, Berlin (1907).
10. Griebsch, A., Zöllner, N.: Verhalten der Harnsäurespiegel im Plasma unter dosierter Zufuhr von Nucleinsäuren. Verh. Dtsch. Ges. inn. Med. **76:** 849 (1970).
11. Griebsch, A., Zöllner, N.: Harnsaure-Plasmaspiegel und renale Harnsäureausscheidung bei Belastung mit Algen, einer purinreichen Eiweißquelle. Verh. Dtsch. Ges. inn. Med. **77:** 173 (1971).

12. Leopold, J.S., Bernhard, A., Jacobi, H.G.: Uric acid metabolism of children. Amer. J. Dis. Childr. **29:** 191 (1925).
13. Löffler, W., Gröbner, W., Medına, R., Zöllner, N.: Untersuchungen des Harnsäurestoffwechsels Gesunder unter oraler Purinbelastung mit Hilfe stabiler Isotopen. Verh. Dtsch. Ges. inn. Med. **86:** 926 (1980a).
14. Löffler, W., Gröbner, W., Zöllner, N.: Influence of dietary protein on serum and urinary uric acid. Adv. Exp. Med. Biol. **122 A:** 209 (1980b).
15. Matzkies, F., Berg, G.: The uricosuric action of amino acids in man. Adv. Exp. Med. Biol. **76 B:** 36 (1977).
16. Nugent, C.A., MacDiarmid, W.D., Tyler, F.H.: Renal excretion of urate in patients with gout. Arch. Intern. Med. **113:** 115 (1964).
17. Nugent, C.A., Tyler, F.H.: The renal excretion of uric acid in patients with gout and in non-gouty subjects. J. Clin. Invest. **38:** 1890 (1959).
18. O'Connor, W.J., Summerill, R.A.: The effect of a meal of meat on glomerular filtration rate in dogs at normal urine flows. J. Physiol. **256:** 81 (1976).
19. Potter, C.F., Cadenhead, A., Sımmonds, H.A., Cameron, J.S.: Differential absorption of purine nucleotides, nucleosides and bases. Adv. Exp. Med. Biol. **122 A:** 203 (1980).
20. Scott, J.T., Pollard, A.C.: Uric acid excretion in the relatives of patients with gout. Ann. Rheum. Dis. **29:** 397 (1970).
21. Seegmiller, J.E., Grayzel, A.J., Laster, L., Lıddle, L.: Uric acıd productıon in gout. J. Clin. Invest. **40:** 1304 (1961).
22. Simmonds, H.A., Hatfield, P.J., Cameron, J.St.: Metabolic studies of purine metabolism in the pig durıng the oral administratıon of guanıne and allopurinol. Biochem. Pharmacol. **22:** 2537 (1973).
23. Spann, W.K., Gröbner, W., Zöllner, N.: Effect of hypoxanthıne ın meat on serum uric acid and urinary urıc acid excretion. Adv. Exp. Med. Bıol. **122 A:** 215 (1980).
24. Taylor, A.E., Rose, W.C.: The ınfluence of protein uptake upon the formation of uric acid. J. Biol. Chem. **18:** 519 (1914).
25. Waslien, C.J., Calloway, D.H., Margen, S.: Uric acid productıon of men fed graded amounts of egg protein and yeast nucleic acid. Amer. J. Clin. Nutr. **21:** 892 (1968).
26. Waslien, C.J., Calloway, D.H., Margen, S., Costa, F.: Uric acid levels in men fed algae and yeast as protein sources. J. Food Sci. **35:** 294 (1970).
27. Wolfson, W.Q., Hunt, H.D., Levine, R., Guterman, H.S., Cohn, C., Rosenberg, E.F., Huddlestun, B., Kadota, K.: The transport and excretion of uric acid ın man. V. A sex difference in urate metabolism. J. Clin. Endocr. **9:** 749 (1949).
28. Yü, T.F., Kaung, C., Gutman, A.B.: Effect of glycine loading on plasma and urinary uric acid and amino acids in normal and gouty subjects. Amer. J. Med. **49:** 352 (1970).
29. Zöllner, N.: Moderne Gichtprobleme. Ätiologie, Pathogenese, Klinik. Ergebn. inn. Med. Kinderheılk. **14:** 21 (1960).
30. Zöllner, N., Grıebsch, A.: Influence of various dıetary purines on uric acid production. In: Urinary caculi. Proceedings of the International Symposium on Renal Stone Research. Madrid, 1972. S. Karger, Basel, 1973.
31. Zöllner, N., Griebsch, A., Gröbner, W.: Einfluß verschiedener Purine auf den Harnsäurestoffwechsel. Ernahrungsumschau **3:** 79 (1972).

Author's address:

Dr. med. W. Löffler
Medızinische Poliklinik der Universität
Pettenkoferstraße 8 a
8000 München 2
Germany

Fortschritte der Urol. und Nephrol. **16**, 19–24 (1981)
Steinkopff Verlag Darmstadt

Mechanisms of Purine Overproduction in Man

William N. Kelley

Department of Internal Medicine, University of Michigan Medical Center
Ann Arbor, USA

Introduction

Several elegant studies conducted first during the 1950s showed that a segment of the gouty population exhibited hyperuricemia as a result of an increased production of uric acid (1,2). Further investigation of this subgroup revealed that these patients also exhibited an accelerated rate of purine biosynthesis *de novo*. In other clinical situation, an increased production of uric acid was noted to result from an accelerated catabolism of purine nucleotides; examples of the latter included the acute leukemias and hemolytic anemias (3–5) where an accelerated turnover of cells leads to an increased degradation of purine nucleotides, thus enhancing uric acid formation. The recognition that the overproduction of uric acid was an important element in the pathophysiology of several clinical conditions provided an incentive to better define mechanisms by which purine biosynthesis was regulated in man. Indeed, the nature of this regulation is now well established and has been reviewed in an earlier paper in this volume (6). In effect, the rate of purine biosynthesis *de novo* (i.e., the pathway leading to the synthesis of inosinic acid from PRPP, glutamine, and other precursors) is tightly controlled by the intracellular concentration of 5-phosphoribosyl-l-pyrophosphate (PRPP) and purine nucleotides (Figure 1). For example, an elevation of the intracellular concentration of PRPP will increase the rate of purine biosynthesis *de novo* while a decrease of the intracellular level of PRPP will decrease the rate of purine biosynthesis *de novo* (7). An increase in the level of the purine nucleoside monophosphates, AMP or GMP, will decrease the rate of purine biosynthesis *de novo* while a decrease in the concentration of these compounds will result in a compensatory increase in purine biosynthesis *de novo* (2). In addition, the level of the purine nucleoside diphosphate, ADP, also appears to play an important role in that increased levels of ADP inhibit PRPP synthetase (8) (Figure 1, reaction 3) and thus reduce levels of PRPP in the cell, hence, reducing the rate of purine biosynthesis de novo. On the other hand, decreased levels of ADP in the cell lead to activation of PRPP synthetase and, thus, increased levels of PRPP in the cell and an accelerated rate of purine synthesis de novo. The molecular alterations of the enzyme PRPP amidotransferase (Figure 1, reaction 1), which nicely account for these observed changes induced by PRPP and purine nucleotides, have been published previcusly (9) and have been summarized in the paper by Dr. Wyngaarden in this volume (6).

It is apparent from the above considerations that an accelerated rate of purine biosynthesis *de novo* can occur, therefore, as a result of either elevated levels of PRPP in the cell or decreased levels of purine nucleotides especially the purine nucleoside monophosphates and ADP. Indeed, it seems likely that in many, if not all, clinical conditions to be described, alterations in the levels of both PRPP and purine nucleotides contribute to the accelerated rate of purine biosynthesis. Despite this prediction, the data currently available would suggest that the intracellular concentration of PRPP ordinarily plays a more important role in accounting for the increased rate of purine biosynthesis than does the reduction of purine nucleotides.

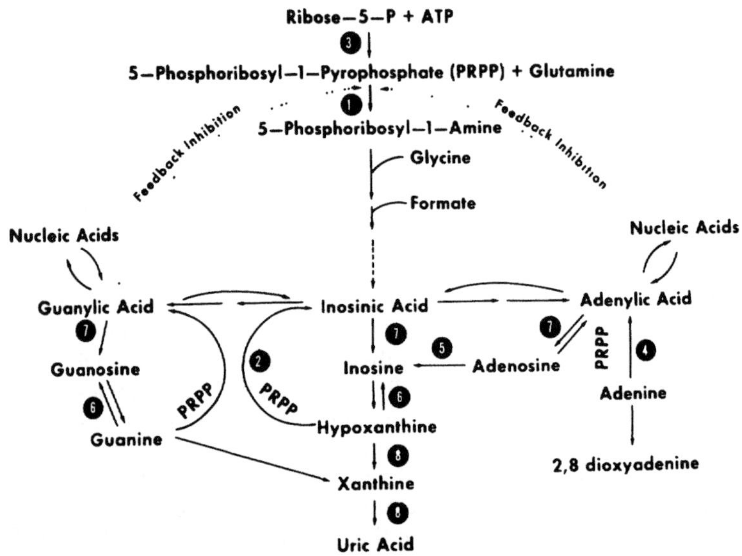

Fig. 1: Outline of purine metabolism. (1) PRPP amidotransferase; (2) hypox Anithine-guanine ribosyltransferase; (3) PRPP synthetase; (4) adenine phosphoribosyltransferse; (5) adenosine de: nase; (6) purine nucleoside phosphorylase; (7) 5'-nucleotidase; (8) xanthine oxidase.

Diseases Associated with Increased Purine Biosynthesis de novo

Hypoxanthine guanine phosphoribosyltransferase deficiency

A deficiency of the enzyme hypoxanthine guanine phosphoribosyltransferase (HPRT) (Figure 1, reaction 2) is associated with two clinical syndromes in man (10,2). The first, described originally by Lesch and Nyhan (11), is characterized by hyperuricemia, a profound overproduction of uric acid, a compulsive desire to self-multilate, choreoathetosis, spasticity, growth and mental retardation as well as a virtually complete deficiency of the enzyme hypoxanthine guanine phosphoribosyltransferase (12). The disease is X-linked and, therefore, occurs in males with transmission through carrier females. A second clinical syndrome associated with a deficiency of the same enzyme was described in 1967 (13). Patients with a partial deficiency of HPRT exhibit hyperuricemia and an overproduction of uric acid but these patients do not go on to exhibit the devastating neurological and behavioral abnormalities characteristic of the Lesch-Nyhan syndrome. In contrast, these patients develop a severe form of gout characterized by onset of joint symptoms occurring often between the ages of 15 and 30, a high incidence of uric acid nephrolithiasis, and, if untreated, a high incidence of tophi (14). All individuals who are either hemizygous or heterozygous for a deficiency of HPRT exhi-

bit an accelerated rate of purine biosynthesis de novo (14). In those hemizygotes who have been carefully studied, this accelerated purine biosynthesis is associated with a striking increase in the intracellular concentration of PRPP with normal levels of purine nucleotides (7). It is thus assumed that the elevated concentration of PRPP in the cell plays a major pathogenetic role in the accelerated rate of purine biosynthesis *de novo* which is observed.
Other factors, however, may also be important. Edwards and co workers (15) have shown that the decreased reutilization of hypoanthine in patients with HPRT deficiency results in the loss of a normal major source of intracellular nucleotide. This drain of hypoxanthine from the cell tends to decrease the consumption of PRPP and reduce the intracellular concentration of IMP. The elevated concentration of PRPP in turn presumably allows the cell to compensate for the loss of IMP by virtue of the accelerated rate of IMP synthesis.

PRPP Synthetase Overactivity

A segment of the gouty population who overproduce uric acid have been shown to have increased activity of the enzyme PRPP synthetase (Figure 1, reaction 3). This disease, which was first described by Sperling and co-workers in 1972 (16), is clinically indistinguishable from that in patients with partial HPRT deficiency. The patients usually have a severe form of gout with a high incidence of uric acid nephrolithiasis and acute gouty arthritis typically occurring before the age of 30. Each patient studied carefully to date has been shown to have an accelerated rate of purine biosynthesis *de novo* as well as elevated levels of PRPP in the cell (17). While the intracellular levels of purine nucleotides have not yet been measured in patients with PRPP synthetase overactivity, it is clear that the elevated levels of PRPP account at least in part for the accelerated rate of purine biosynthesis observed in these patients.
The elevated levels of PRPP found in patients with this disease are presumed to result from an increased formation of PRPP rather than from the decreased degradation of this compound.

Other Types of Gout

The presence of both HPRT deficiency and PRPP synthetase overactivity accounts for only a small fraction of gouty patients who are overproducers of uric acid. Becker has studied cultured cells derived from seven patients with gout who were overproducers and had elevated levels of PRPP in fibroblasts but had neither HPRT deficiency nor PRPP synthetase overactivity. In two of these cases he has found elevated intracellular levels of ribose-5-phosphate and an increased rate of PRPP generation providing evidence to suggest an acceleration in the hexose monophosphate shunt in these patients leading to the elevated levels of ribose-5-phosphate. The possibility exists in these two patients that the elevated levels of ribose-5-phosphate would in turn lead to elevated levels of PRPP and, hence, to the accelerated rate of purine biosynthesis. The exact mechanism responsible for the elevated levels of ribose-5-phosphate, however, has not been established nor have the intracellular levels of purine nucleotides been measured in cells from this group of patients.

Purine Nucleoside Phosphorylase Deficiency

In 1975, Giblett and co-workers (18) described a deficiency of the enzyme purine nucleoside phosphorylase in patients with severe combined immunodeficiency disease characterized clinically by a severe abnormality of T-lymphocyte function. While these patients often exhibit hypouricemia as a result of the deficiency of purine nucleoside phosphorylase, they exhibit at the same time accelerated levels of purine biosynthesis *de novo* with increased excretion of adenosine, deoxyinosine, guanosine, and deoxyguanosine (19). In addition, the intracellular levels of PRPP are elevated in patients with purine nucleoside phosphorylase deficiency. It is assumed, therefore, that the accelerated rate of purine biosynthesis may be due, at least in part, to the elevated levels of PRPP. It has been suggested that a decreased availability of the substrates hypoxanthine and guanine leads to a decreased functional activity of the enzyme HPRT thus leading to decreased consumption of PRPP and hence the elevated levels observed.

Pharmocologic Alterations of purine Biosynthesis de novo

A number of compounds are capable of altering the rate of purine biosynthesis *de novo*. Many that are capable of inhibiting purine biosynthesis *de novo* appear to do so as a result of depletion of intracellular levels of PRPP (7). In most of these cases, the nucleotide derivative of the compound is formed and this derivative may also play a role in the inhibition of the PRPP amidotransferase and/or PRPP synthetase. Examples include adenine, allopurinol, 2'6-diaminopurine, nicotinic acid, and orotic acid. On the other hand, several compounds have been studied which lead to an acceleration in the rate of purine biosynthesis apparently mediated by an increased level of PRPP (7). Examples of this category might include fructose, methylene blue, ACTH, TSH, and estrogens.

Conditions Associated with Increased Degradation of purine Nucleotides

An increased production of uric acid can result from clinical conditions in which there is a rapid increase in the rate of degradation of purine nucleotides. This degradation occurs as a result of the turnover or breakdown of nucleic acids and soluble nucleotides in the cell often associated with breakdown of the cell itself. Examples of this would include the acute leukemias and hemolytic anemias (2). In addition, the degradation of purine nucleotides can occur as a result of alterations in the energy of the cell which enhance the breakdown of ATP. Examples of this might include starvation, muscular exertion, and hypoxia. In some of these latter conditions related to the catabolism of purine nucleoside triphosphates, there may also be compensatory increase in the rate or purine biosynthesis *de novo* related to the release of feedback inhibition at the level of PRPP synthetase and/or PRPP amidotransferase.

Conclusion

In summary, the overproduction of purines in man may be related to a primary abnormality leading to an accelerated rate of purine biosynthesis *de novo* or to a degradation of purine nucleotides and nucleic acids. An accelerated rate of purine biosynthesis *de novo* could occur as a result of either an increased level of PRPP in the cell or a decrease in the concentration of purine nucleotides. Clinically, an elevated concentration of PRPP appears to be the primary mechanism responsible for the accelerated rate of purine biosynthesis in most conditions associated with this abnormality which have been carefully investigated in man. PRPP levels may be increased because of an increased rate of synthesis as occurs in patients with PRPP synthetase overactivity or as a result of a decreased rate of degradation as occurs classically in patients with a deficiency of hypoxanthine guanine phosphoribosyltransferase.

References

1. Benedict, J.D., Roche, M., Yu, T.-F., Bien, E.G., Gutman, A.B., and Stetten, D., Jr.: Incorporation of glycine nitrogen into uric acid in normal and gouty man. Metabolism, **1:** 3, 1952.
2. Wyngaarden, J.B. and Kelley, W.N.: Gout in *The Metabolic Basis of Inherited Diseases,* 4th ed., edited by Stanbury, J.B., Wyngaarden, J.B. and Fredrickson, D.S., McGraw-Hill Book Co., New York, 1978, pp. 1045–1071.
3. Bishop, C., Garner, W., and Talbott, J.H.: Pool size, turnover rate, and rapidity of equilibration of injected isotopic uric acid in normal and pathological subjects. J. Clin. Invest., **30:** 879, 1951.
4. Yu, T.-F., Weissmann, B., Sharney, L., Kupfer, S., and Gutman, A.B.: On the biosynthesis of uric acid from glycine- NS in primary and secondary polycythemia. Am. J. Med.,·**21:** 901, 1956.
5. Laster, L., and Muller, A.F.: Uric acid production in a case of myeloid metaplasia associated with gouty arthritis, studied with N^{15}-labeled glycine. Am. J. Med., **15:** 857, 1953.
6. Wyngaarden, J.B.: Paper in this symposium.
7. Fox, I., and Kelley, W.N.: Phosphoribosylpyrophosphate (PRPP) in man: Biochemical and Clinical significance. Ann. Intern. Med., **74:** 424, 1971.
8. Fox, I.H., and Kelley, W.N.: Human phosphoribosyl-pryrophosphate synthetase: Kinetic mechanism and end-product inhibition. J. Biol. Chem. **247:** 2126, 1972.
9. Holmes, E.W., Wyngaarden, J.B., and Kelley, W.N.: Human glutamine phosphoribosylpyrophosphate amidotransferase: Two molecular forms interconvertible by purine ribonucleotides and phosphoribosylpyrophosphate. J. Biol. Chem., **248:** 6035, 1973.
10. Kelley, W.N. and Wyngaarden, J.B.: The Lesch-Nyhan Syndrome in *The Metabolic Basis of Inherited Diseases,* 4th ed., edited by Stanbury, J.B., Wyngaarden, J.B., and Fredrickson, D.S., Mc-Graw-Hill Book Co., New York, 1978, pp. 916–1010.
11. Lesch, M., and Nyhan, W.L.: A familial disorder of uric acid metabolism and central nervous system function. Am. J. Med. **36:** 561, 1964.
12. Seegmiller, J.E.; Rosenbloom, R.M., and Kelley, W.N.: An enzyme defect associated with a sex-linked human neurological disorder and excessive purine synthesis. Science, **155:** 1682, 1967.
13. Kelley, W.N., Rosenbloom, F.M., Henderson, J.F., and Seegmiller, J.E.: A specific enzyme defect in gout associated with overproduction of uric acid. Proc. Natl. Acad. Sci. USA, **57:** 1735, 1967.
14. Kelley, W.N., Greene, M.L., Rosenbloom, F.M., Henderson, J.F., and Seegmiller, J.E.: Hypoxanthine-guanine phosphoribosyltransferase deficiency in gout. Ann. Intern. Med.. **70:** 155, 1969.
15. Edwards, N.L., Recker, D., and Fox, I.H.: Overproduction of uric acid in hypoxanthine-guanine phosphoribosyltransferase deficiency: Contribution by impaired purine salvage. J. Clin. Inves., **63:** 922–930, 1979.
16. Sperling, O., Eilam, G., Persky-Broxh, S., and DeVries, A.: Accelerated erythrocyte 5-phosphoribosyl-l-pyrophosphate synthesis: A familial abnormality associated with excessive uric acid production and gout. Biochem. Med., **6:** 310, 1972.
17. Wyngaarden, J.B. and Kelley, W.N.: Gout with purine overproduction due to increased phosphoribosylpyrophosphate synthetase activity. In **Gout and Hyperuricemia,** Chapter 24, Grune & Stratton, New York, 1976, pp. 301–308.
18. Giblett, E.R., Ammann, A.J., Wara, D.W., Sandman, R., and Diamond, L.K.: Nucleoside-phosphorylase deficiency in a child with severely defective T-cell immunity and normal B-cell immunity. Lancet, **I:** 1010–3, 1975.

19. Cohen, A., Doyle, D., Martin, D.W., Jr., and Ammann, A.J.: Abnormal purine metabolism and purine overproduction in a patient deficient in purine nucleoside phosphorylase. N. Engl. J. Med., 295: 1449–54, 1976.

Author's address:

Prof. Dr. *W.N. Kelley*
University of Michigan
Medical School
Dept. Internal Medicine
Ann Arbor, Mi 48109
USA

Fortschritte der Urol. und Nephrol. **16**, 25–31 (1981)
Steinkopff Verlag Darmstadt

Uric Acid Hyperproduction and Isohydric Steady-state in Gouty Patients

P. Leskovar, R. Hartung, A. Siebert, and E. Wellnhofer

Urologische Klinik und Poliklinik rechts der Isar der Technischen Universität München, West Germany

1. Introduction

The interrelation between overproduced uric acid and the acid–base balance in gouty patients should be discussed from the chemical, biochemical, and clinical points of view.

Firstly, the influence of main dietary representants, the carbohydrates, the fats, and the proteins on the acid–base balance should be mentioned. In addition, the function of the biosynthesized uric acid on the alkali reserve will be discussed in some detail. Subsequently, some quantitative aspects of uric acid synthesis, turnover, and renal and extrarenal excretion in healthy persons and gouty patients will be dealt with, followed by the detailed description of a special mechanism, preserving the serum bicarbonate by mobilization of bone phosphates. Finally, some clinical observations, supporting our conception of the interrelation between hyperproduced uric acid and acid-base balance, will be discussed briefly.

As is well known, the dietary carbohydrates are normally catabolized to give the neutral end products carbon dioxide and water. The intermediately formed organic acids such as lactic acid or tri- and dicarbonic acids of the Krebs cycle solely influence the acid-base balance if they are excreted in their ionic form, leaving behind the protons that would normally be oxidized together with the acidic anion to the neutral end products mentioned above. The same is true for the fatty acids, originating from the dietary fats. Under special circumstances, the fatty acid degradation leads to the accumulation of ketone bodies. The excretion of acetoacetic and of β-hydroxybutyric acid in their ionic form results in acidosis, as observed in diabetes. Under normal conditions, however, there is no influence of dietary fat on the acid-base balance.

In the case of dietary proteins, the sulfur-containing amino acids such as cysteine and methionine lead to the formation of sulfuric acid that dissociates to protons and sulfate and strongly loads the plasma bicarbonate. The pulmonal and renal defense mechanisms successfully prevent acidosis, however. The dietary proteins are primarily responsible for the low pH values of urine, compared with plasma.

In general, it can be stated that acids, applied as acids or synthesized endogenously, do not influence the acid–base balance if they are eliminated unchanged as acids. However, they exert a clear influence on the plasma bicarbonate if they are excreted, renally or extrarenally, in the ionized form as anions, leaving their proton behind in the extracellular fluid. Examples of exogenously applicable, urine acidifying substances are hydrochloric and phosphoric acid, ammonium chloride, lysine and glutamine hydrochloride, and calcium chloride. The two mineral acids are excreted as chloride and phosphate anions, respectively. The ammonium ion of ammonium chloride is eliminated as neutral urea and the chloride ion as an anion, leaving behind in sum a proton in the extracellular fluid. The two amino acids in lysine and glutamine hydrochloride are metabolized, leaving behind the urine-acidifying hydrochloride in blood. Calcium chloride is urine acidifying because of the partial binding of Ca on phosphate, oxalate, and fatty acids, with resulting release of hydrochloride.

Examples of endogenously formed, acid–base-balance-influencing acids and/or endogenously formed urine-acidifying acids are overproduced lactic, acetoacetic, ,-hydroxybutyric and, uric acids. The latter will be discussed in some detail.

2. De novo Synthesis of uric acid

As is well known, the two purines, adenine and guanine, originating from nucleic acids or from high-energy phosphate compounds like ATP or GTP, are catabolized in man to uric acid. The intermediately formed hypoxanthine and xanthine are both oxidized to uric acid by the enzyme xanthine oxidase. This enzyme introduces an oxygen atom between the carbon and hydrogen atom in position C_8. Of the two tautomeric forms of uric acid, the amido (lactam) and the imido (lactim) forms, the latter has a more acid character.

Uric acid is not a "typical" organic acid: the acidic properties do not stem from a dissociation of a carboxylic or sulfonic groups but from a proton dissociation of the purine ring.

The reported pK_1 values range from 3.9 to 5.7 (21, 48). For our considerations it is essential that the pK value of uric acid is lower than that of bicarbonate, the latter being 6.1. All acids with a pK value of less than 6.1 are able to release carbon dioxide from bicarbonate. Our gasometric measurements showed a slow but clear release of carbon dioxide after addition of uric acid to sodium bicarbonate. A prolonged overproduction of acids (even weak acids such as uric acid inevitably impairs the alkali reserve if this is not compensated for.

It must be underlined however, that the daily de-novo-synthetized (not absolute) concentration of uric acid is responsible for the acid load. In the presence of tophi, one must further take into account that the monosodium urate, deposited in tophi (20), has been formed by leaving behind in extracellular fluid an equivalent amount of hydrogen ions.

3. Uric acid in Healthy persons and gouty Patients: Miscible pool and Turnover

The miscible urate pool in normal male subjects is 866 to 1587 mg (mean 1200 mg) (38, 41, 51, 2, 11, 4, 5, 52, 22). Scott (37) reported values of between 992 and 1650 mg (mean 1221). In female healthy persons, the miscible urate pool is considerably lower (541 to 687 mg, mean 614 mg) (52, 22). In gouty patients, the miscible urate pool is markedly increased (2000–4000 mg) (38). Scott (37) found values of 1248 to 3199 mg and a mean of 2027 mg in his patients. Other investigators reported values as high as 3000–5000 mg (2, 4). In patients with tophaceous gout, the miscible urate pool can reach values of 18 000–31 000 mg (3). Following Sorensen's estimations the amount of urate in the tophaceous compartment that was participating in a slow exchange with the soluble urate of plasma was around 300 times the size of the miscible pool (43). In healthy subjects 45–85% (mean 60%) of the urate pool is daily renewed (17). The average daily urate turnover is 602–838 mg (mean 701 mg) (37) and 513–1108 mg (mean 695 mg) (41, 30). In gouty patients without tophi, the urate turnover amounts to 506–1542 mg (mean 861 mg) (37). In patients with tophaceous gout, the urate turnover is around 50% of the miscible pool (29). Extreme values are as high as 96% (4). In patients with Lesch-Nyhan syndrome the daily urate turnover is around 200% of the miscible pool (24).

4. Renal and Extrarenal urate Excretion

In normal subjects, a daily uric acid excretion of 80 to 976 mg (50) was reported. At a purine reach diet healthy persons can excrete up to 2000 mg uric acid daily (50). Patients with idiopathic gout show a wide range of values to over 1500 mg per day. The extrarenal uric acid excretion must be considerable because only 55–95% (mean 75%) of intravenously given uric acid appeared in urine (41, 42, 11, 5, 52). Sorensen (41) estimated the gastrointestinally eliminated uric acid as 200 mg, corresponding to 1/3 of the urate turnover. In gouty patients the extrarenally excreted uric acid is absolutely and relatively increased so that only 35--54% of the uric acid appeared in urine (22, 39). The increased extrarenal urate elimination could be the consequence of the impaired renal function. Sorensen (45) showed that patients with high grade renal failure excrete up to 70% of uric acid extrarenally.

5. Mechanisms of renal acid Elimination

5.1 Tubular Secretion of hydrogen Ions

Essentially, the suggested mechanism includes metabolic production of carbon dioxide, hydration to carbonic acid, catalysis by carbonic anhydrase, dissociation of carbonic acid, and exchange of the hydrogen ions for sodium ions across the luminal border of the cell.

5.2 Binding of Excreted Hydrogen ions on secondary Phosphate in urine

Around one-third of the excreted hydrogen ions are bound to secondary phosphate ions, preventing depletion of plasma bicarbonate in this way.

5.3 Ammonia Excretion

The tubular glutaminase releases free ammonia from glutamine. After diffusion into the tubular lumen, ammonia combines with hydrogen ions to the physiologically neutral ammonium ion which replaces the sodium ion in urine and preserves the plasma bicarbonate.

5.4 Elimination of surplus Hydrogen ions by Undissociated acids

Organic acids like lactic, pyruvic, di- and tricarboxylic acids of the Krebs cycle, and uric acid, which contribe essentially to the titratable acidity of urine, can at low urinary pH combine with excreted hydrogen ions and prevent depletion of the alkali reserve in this way.

5.5 Mobilization of bone Phosphates and Substitution of Bone-Derived Calcium ions for Sodium ions in Urine

One additional mechanism is available for combating acidosis, being of significance especially in prolonged (latent) acidoses. This is the substitution of calcium ions for sodium ions in urine. The source of this calcium is the bone material, which increases in solubility with decreasing pH. As tertiary phosphate, $Ca_3(PO_4)_2$, from bone enters plasma, it reacts with the carbonic acid (H_2CO_3): $3\,Ca^{2+} + 2\,PO_4^{3-} + 2\,H_2CO_3 \rightarrow 3\,Ca^{2+} + 2\,HPO_4^{2-} + 2\,HCO_3^-$

The bicarbonate (HCO_3^-) ions formed are available to neutralize two molecules of an acid with a pK less than the pK of carbonic acid (H_2CO^3), e.g., de-novo-synthesized uric acid.

$2\,HCO_3^- + 2\,HA \rightarrow 2\,H_2CO_3 + 2\,A^-$

so that the mixture in plasma may be considered to be the following:

$3\,Ca^{2+} + 2\,HPO_4^{2-} + 2\,A^-$

Addition of a second pair of acid molecules to the plasma and their reaction with bicarbonate give the following:

$2\,Na^+ + 2\,HCO_3^- + 2\,HA \rightarrow 2\,Na^+ + 2\,A^- + 2\,H_2CO_3$

The total mixture presented to the glomerulus is then $2\,Na^+, 4\,A^-, 3\,Ca^{2+}$, and $2\,HPO_4^{2-}$.

If the usual acidification device is operative,

$2\,Na^+ + 2\,HPO_4^{2-} + 2\,H_2CO_3 \rightarrow 2\,Na^+$ (plasma) $+ 2\,HCO_3^-$ (plasma) $+ 2\,H_2PO_4^-$ (urine)

The overall reaktion, then, is:

$3\,Ca^{2+} + 2\,HPO_4^{2-} + 4\,HA \rightarrow 3\,Ca^{2+} + 2\,H_2PO_4^- + 4\,A^-$

and 1 mole of tricalciumphosphate, $Ca_3(PO_4)_2$, makes possible the excretion of 4 equivalents of acid. This represents an extremely effective mechanism for preventing depletion of the alkali reserve, although it may result ultimately in serious bone demineralization.

Analogous equations for hydroxylapatite, $Ca_3(PO_4)_2 \cdot Ca(OH)_2$, and for carbonate apatite, $3Ca_3(PO_4)_2 \cdot CaCO_3 \cdot H_2O$, are known, but can not be presented here.

Uric acid, if prolongedly overproduced, fulfils all the criteria of such an acid: the pK value is less than that of bicarbonate and dissociation at the pH of extracellular fluid is nearly 100%. Quantitatively, uric acid is one of the main urinary organic acids. Daily molar excretion of uric acid is 0.47 to 5.80 and is comparable to that of citric acid (0.47–4.34), lactic acid (0.76–4.54), and ketone bodies (0.10–0.97). On average, 50–90% of urinary urate is in ionic form and loads to this extent the isohydry.

6. Clinical Observations indirectly supporting our Conception

Gutman and Yü (18) reported that gouty patients surprisingly often form Ca stones, especially the Ca oxalate calculi. Several investigators (19, 40, 31, 9, 26, 14, 36) have underlined the coincidence of increased uric acid level in blood and/or urine and Ca oxalate lithiasis. Coe (6) observed a parallelism between hyperuricosuria and idiopathic hypercalciuria. He also reproted the successful therapy of Ca oxalate nephrolithiasis by the uricostaticum allopurinol (7). Schwille et al. (34) found out that patients with urate calculi as well as those with hypercalciuria tend to have a parathormone-independent phosphate loss in urine. In another paper (35), Schwille reported increased chloride and decreased bicarbonate in the plasma of urate stone formers, which can only be explained by a (latent) acidosis in these patients. Comar and Bronner (8) discussed increased calcium and magnesium excretion, accompanying the raised urinary excretion of organic acids (uric acid).

In addition, radiologic studies (13, 12, 10, 33) give evidence of bone demineralization in tophaceous gout. As bone demineralization up to 30% (1) remains unperceived and the function of highly demineralized bones must not be impaired (32), the acidosis preventing mobilization of bone material in tophaceous gout can proceed latently.

Our own measurements of uric acid and calcium in the morning, midday, and evening urinary samples of 10 oxalate stone formers and 11 controls during a period of 4–6 weeks showed a high positive correlation in the group of recurrent stone formers, the coefficient of correlation(r) being 0.85 and the corresponding linear regression: Ca = 1.54 x uric acid – 0.14; in the group of controls, the correlation was moderate, the coefficient of correlation amounting to 0.44 and the equation for the linear regression being: Ca = 0.79 x uric acid + 1.31.

An additional observation, hinting indirectly at the parallelism between uric acid and calcium in urine, is the high coincidence of uric acid and calcium crystalluria in the group of recurrent stone formers that has been measured in 16 (oxalate and urate) stone patients and in 11 controls during our long-term study. Twenty-eight percent of all urine samples collected in male stone patients and thirty-one percent of those collected in female patients contained both calcium and uric acid crystals.

References

1. Babaianth, L.: Radiol.clin. (Basel) **16:** 291 (1947).
2. Benedict, J.D., P.H. Forsham, De W. Stetten jr.: J. Biol. Chem. **181:** 183 (1949).
3. Benedict, J.D., P.H. Forsham, M. Roche, S. Soloway, De W. Stetten Jr.: J. clin. Invest. **29:** 1104 (1950).
4. Bishop, C., W. Garner, J.H. Talbott: J. Clin. Invest. **30:** 879 (1951).
5. Buzard, J., C. Bishop, J.H. Tabott: J. Biol. Chem. **196:** 179 (1952).
6. Coe, F.L.: Clin. Res. **20:** 589 (1972).
7. Coe, F.L., L. Raisen: The Lancet, January 20 (1973) p. 129.
8. Comar, C.L., F. Bronner: Mineral Metabolism, An Advanced Treatise. Vol. III (Calcium Physiology). Academic Press, New York–London 1969
9. Dent, C.E., D.J. Sutor: Lancet (1971) 775.
10. Dihlmann, W., H.J. Fernholz: Dtsch. med. Wschr. **94:** 1909 (1969).
11. Geren, W., A. Bendich, O. Bodansky, G.B. Brown: J. Biol. Chem. **183:** 21 (1950).
12. Golding, D.N.: Rheumatische Erkrankungen. Thieme Verlag, Stuttgart 1967.
13. Grafe, E.: Ernahrungs- und Stoffwechselkrankheiten. In: Lehrbuch der Inneren Medizin, Bd. II, 6. u. 7. Aufl. hrsg. v. H. Schwiegle und A. Jores. Springer-Verlag, Berlin 1949.
14. Grob, K.U., K. Bandhauer: Vortrag auf Bonn–Wiener–Harnsteinsymposium, Wien 1973.
15. Gutman, A.B., T.F. Yü: Amer. J. Med. **23:** 600–622 (1957).
16. Gutman, A.B., T.F. Yu: Amer. J. Med. **35:** 820 (1963).
17. Gutman, A.B., T.F. Yu: New Engl. J. Med. **273:** 313 (1965).

18. Gutman, A.B., T.F. Yü: Amer. J. Med. **45:** 756 (1968).
19. Hartung, R.: Münch. med. Wschr. **117/10:** 387 (1975).
20. Howell, R.R., E.D. Eanes, J.E. Seegmiller: Arthr. and Rheum. **6:** p. 97 (1963).
21. Klages, F.: Lehrbuch der organischen Chemie. Bd. III, 2. neubearbeitete Aufl., S. 490–496. W. de Gruyter & Co., Berlin 1967.
22. Kelley, W.N., F.M. Rosenbloom, J.E. Seegmiller, R.R. Howell: J. Pediat. **72:** 488 (1968).
23. Leskovar, P., R. Hartung: Therapiewoche **27:** 1152–1156 (1977).
24. Lesch, M., W.L. Nyhan: Amer. J. Med. **36:** 561 (1964).
25. Lucke, H.: Z. Ges. exp. Med. **76:** 188 (1931).
26. Lutzeyer, W., B. Terhorst: Jenaer Harnsteinsymposium 1972, S. 191. Wiss. Beiträge der Universität Jena.
27. Mertz, D.P.: Dtsch. med. J. **19:** 413 (1968).
28. Mertz, D.P.: Gicht, Grundlagen, Klinik und Therapie. 2. Aufl., S. 213. Georg Thieme Verlag, Stuttgart 1973.
29. Mertz, D.P.: Gicht, Grundlagen, Klinik und Therapie. 2. Aufl., S. 334. Georg Thieme Verlag, Stuttgart 1973.
30. Miller, C.S., S. Gurin, D.W. Wilson: Science **112:** 654 (1950).
31. Prien, E.L., E.L. Prien jr.: Amer. J. Med. **45:** 654 (1968).
32. Raaflaub, J.: Schweiz. med. Wschr. **48:** 1417 (1961).
33. Schacherl, M., F. Schilling, A. Gamp: Radiologe **6:** 231 (1966).
34 Schwille, P.O., U. Jügelt, A. Sigel: Der Urologe **A 11:** 185–189 (1972).
35. Schwille, P.O.: Urin-pH, Titrationsazidität, Ammonium und einige organische Sauren (Harnsäure, Zitrat, Kreatinin) bei Nierensteinkranken, in: Pathogenese und Klinik der Harnsteine II, 2. Symposium in Bonn am 24. und 25. 11. 1972 (Hrsg.: W. Vahlensieck und G. Gasser), S. 123–126. Dr. D. Steinkopff Verlag, Darmstadt 1974.
36. Schwille, P.O.: Therapiewoche **26:** 5900–5906 (1976).
37. Scott, J.T., V.P. Holloway, H.I. Glass, R.N.: Ann. Rheum. Dis. **28:** 366 (1969).
38. Seegmiller, J.E., A.I. Grayzel, L. Laster, L. Liddle: J. Clin. Invest. **40:** 1304 (1961).
39. Skupp, S., J.H. Ayvazian: J. Lab. clin. Med. **73:** 909 (1969).
40. Smith, M.J.V.: J. Urol. (Baltimore) **101:** 637 (1969).
41. Sorensen, L.B.: Metabolism. **8:** 687 (1959).
42. Sorensen, L.B.: Scand. J. clin Lab. Invest. **12:** supp 54 (1960)
43. Sorensen, L.B.: Arch. Intern. Med. (Chicago) **109:** 379 (1962)
44. Sorensen, L.B.: Med. Clin. N. Amer. **47:** 169 (1963).
45. Sorensen, L.B.: Arthr. and Rheum. **8:** 694 (1965).
46. Talbott, J.H., K.L. Terplan: Medicine **39:** 405 (1960).
47. Vogler, W.R., J.W. Drane: Metabolism **18:** 519 (1969).
48. White, A., P. Handler, E.L. Smith: Principles of Biochemistry. Fifth edition, p. 183. McGraw-Hill Koagakusha Ltd., Tokyo–Düsseldorf 1973.
49. White, A., P. Handler, E.L. Smith: ibid., p. 999
50. Wissenschaftliche Tabellen, 7. Aufl., S. 667. Documenta Geigy (Redaktion: K. Diem und C. Lentner). J.R. Geigy AG, Pharma, Basel.
51. Wyngaarden, J.B., D. Stetten jr.: J. Biol. Chem. **203:** 9 (1953).
52. Wyngaarden, J.B.: J. Clin. Invest. **34:** 256 (1955).
53. Zöllner, N.: Z. klin. Chem. **1:** 178 (1963).
54. Zöllner, N.: Dtsch. med. Wschr. **93:** 310 (1968).

General Literature

1. Christensen, H.N.: Elektrolytstoffwechsel, Springer-Verlag, Berlin–Heidelberg–New York 1969
2. Davenport, H.W.: Saure-Basen-Regulation. G. Thieme Verlag, Stuttgart 1973
3. Deetjen, P., J.W. Boylan, K. Kramer: Niere und Wasserhaushalt, 2. Aufl., in: Gauer-Kramer-Jung: Physiologie des Menschen VII. Urban & Schwarzenberg, München–Berlin–Wien 1973
4. Hills, G.A.: Acid-Base Balance, Chemistry, Physiology, Pathophysiology. The Williams & Wilkins Company, Baltimore 1973

5. Muntrogler, E.: Elektrolytstoffwechsel und Säure-Basen-Gleichgewicht. W. de Gryter Verlag, Berlin–New York 1973
6. Truniger, B.: Wasser- und Elektrolythaushalt, Diagnostik und Therapie, 4. überarb. Aufl. G. Thieme Verlag, Stuttgart 1974.

Author's address:

Dr. *Peter Leskovar*
Biochemisches Forschungslabor
der Urologischen Klinik und Poliklinik
rechts der Isar der TU München
8000 München 80
Ismaningerstr. 22
Germany

Fortschritte der Urol. und Nephrol. 16, 32–35 (1981)
Steinkopff Verlag Darmstadt

Juvenile Gout and Hyperuricosuria Due to Chronic Compensated Hemolytic Syndrome

U. A. Liberman, R. Samuel, A. Halabe, and O. Sperling

Metabolic unit and Department of Clinical Biochemistry, Beilinson Medical Center, Tel-Aviv University School of Medicine, Petah-Tikva, Israel

In recent years it has become evident that the proportion of purine overproducers among the gouty population is smaller than was previously estimated (1). In addition, the reason for purine overproduction in most of the overproducing patients is still unknown. Only in a limited number could a hereditary enzymatic defect be proved (2). Recently we found a patient with juvenile gout due to chronic compensated (nonanemic) intracorpuscular hemolysis. In a subsequent study of our gouty patients suspected of being overproducers (urinary urate excretion on a regular home diet > 900 mg/24 h), an additional 7 patients, representing a substantial proportion of all our purine-overproducing gouty patients, were found with evidence suggesting the presence of chronic compensated hemolysis. It thus appears that chronic compensated hemolysis may be a relatively common cause of metabolic gout.
In this communication we present the case report of the patient with juvenile gout due to chronic compensated hemolytic syndrome as well as data presently available on the other patients suspected of being similarly affected.

Case report

The patient, a 53-year-old male, started to suffer from recurrent attacks, resembling gouty arthritis, at the age of 14 years. At the age of 21, the diagnosis of gout was made, based on the demonstration of sodium urate crystals in biopsy material obtained from a tophus in one of his toes and on the finding of hyperuricemia (blood urate 9 mg/dl). In the following years, the frequency of the arthritis attacks increased, spreading to his elbows, toes, and fingers. At the age of 33, the patient was referred to our attention. On admission his blood urate was 15.2 mg/dl and his urinary uric acid excretion ranged from 1293 to 1540 mg/24 h. All other routine laboratory tests were normal. The patient was treated by probenecid as well as by alkalinization to prevent uric acid lithiasis. For the next 5 years, urinary urate excretion ranged from 1320 to 2400 mg/24 h while his blood urate level ranged from 7.3 to 11. 3 mg/dl. In 1965 allopurinol treatment was begun and the uric acid level in his blood and urine decreased to the normal range.
No evidence for the presence of a known enzyme abnormality causing purine overproduction could be obtained. The erythrocyte activity of hypoxanthine-guanine phosphoribosyltransferase (HGPRT), of adenine phosphoribosyltransferase (APRT), and of phosphoribosylpyrophosphate (PRPP) synthetase were all in the normal range. Erythrocyte PRPP generation, as well as the acitivity of the pentose phosphate pathway was also normal (Table 1). In addition, the rate of de novo synthesis of purine nucleotides in cultured skin fibroblasts from the patient was found to be normal.

Table 1: Erythrocyte parameters of purine metabolism

Parameter	Subjects Control		Patient
HGPRT*	96.8 ±	10.1	98.2
APRT*	28.4 ±	5.8	31.3
PRPP synthetase*	15.1 ±	2.8	19.5
Adenine incorporation**	1.51 ±	0.29	1.53
PRPP generation**	1.55 ±	0.28	1.17
Oxidative pentose shunt***	514.0	± 160	662.0

* nmol/mg protein/h
** nmol/ml packed cells/min
*** nmol/g Hb/h

Table 2: Indices of hemolysis

Hemoglobin	14– 15%
Reticulocyte count	22–100‰
Serum bilirubin (total)	1.5–4.9 mg/dl
Serum bilirubin (indirect)	0.9–3.8 mg/dl
Serum haptoglobin	0– 50 mg/dl
Serum iron	130–230 μg/dl
Urinary iron	7.6 mg/24 h
Fecal stercobilinogen	539–963 mg/24 h

Table 3: Ferrokinetic studies

Parameter	Patient	Normal
Plasma clearance half-life (months)	32	60–90
Plasma turnover (mg%/24 h)	4.56	1
Incorporation into erythrocytes (% in 10 days)	100	80

In 1968, laboratory tests carried out to clarify the reason for the appearance of a mild jaundice demonstrated the presence of compensated hemolysis (Table 2). The diagnosis of hemolysis was based on the following: constant presence of elevated serum indirect bilirubin, very low level to complete absence of haptoglobin, high reticulocyte count, high serum and urinary iron levels, and markedly abnormal ferrokinetics (Table 3), as well as elevated plasma hemoglobin and fecal stercobilinogen. The additional finding of a negative Coombs test, and of a markedly shortened half-life of the patients erythrocytes in contrast to a normal half-life of erythrocytes from a healthy donor in the same patient (Table 4), demonstrated the intracorpuscular nature of the hemolysis. All tests performed so far, which were aimed to identify the erythrocyte abnormality causing the intracorpuscular hemolysis, including the mechanical and osmotic fragility of the erythrocytes, hemoglobin electrophoresis, and erythrocyte enzymes profile, have given results within the normal range.

A study of the patients family revealed low haptoglobin values in only the patients son. This finding suggests hereditary recessive pattern.

Table 4: Erythrocyte half-life

Patients erythrocytes	11 days
Normal donor erythrocytes in patients circulation	25 days
Normal erythrocates	28 ± 3 days

Based on this experience, all gouty patients with suspected purine overproduction not due to hereditary enzyme abnormalities were evaluated for the presence of compensated hemolysis. So far, 7 patients have been found in which the serum haptoglobin level was indicative of hemolysis (Table 5). In 5 of these patients, a shortened erythrocyte half-life was also found.

Table 5: Patients with hyperuricemia and hyperuricosuria due to compensated hemolysis

Patient	Uric acid*				
	serum mg/dl	urine mg/24 h	Clinical manifestation	Haptoglobin (mg/dl)	RBC half-life (days)
1	7.8–7.9	740– 992		0–45	20
2	7.4–7.9	600– 884	nephrolithiasis	0–40	21
3.	7.5–8.4	800– 900	nephrolithiasis	0–35	20
4.	8.7–9.6	800–1113	nephrolithiasis and gout	0–70	
5	7.6–8.0	800– 900		0–10	17
6	8.4–9.4	900– 940	gout	25	19.5
7	8.6–9.6	900–1100	gout	30–50	

* Values obtained on a regular home diet.

Discussion

The patient described represents a case in which the symptomatology and biochemical findings compatible with juvenile primary metabolic gout were later found to be the manifestations of secondary metabolic gout, due to a chronic compensated hemolytic syndrome of an as yet unkown etiology. The finding of additional 7 gouty purine-overproducing patients with laboratory data indicating the presence of compensated hemolysis suggests that such syndromes may be a more common cause for uric acid overproduction then was previously estimated. Indeed, gout due to hemolytic anemia has been described before in several conditions (3–7). However, as a presenting symptom of nonanemic, well-compensated hemolytic conditions, it has not yet been reported. Since hyperuricosuria is a major potential cause for uric acid lithiasis, the role of chronic compensated hemolytic syndromes in stone formation should be taken into consideration.

References

1. Wyngaarden, J.B.: Adv. Exp. Med. & Biol. **76B:** 361, 1977.
2. Wyngaarden, J.B.: Gout, in The Metabolic Basis of Inherited Disease, Stanbury, J.B. Wyngaarden, J.B., Fredrickson, D.S., Editors, McGraw-Hill, N.Y. 1978, P-916.

3. Wacker, B.R. and Alexander, F.: J.A.M.A. **215:** 255, 1971.
4. Spivack, M., Gold, M., Williams, J.C. and Graw, V.: J.A.M.A. **206:** 1572, 1968.
5. Ball, G.V. and Sorensen, L.B.: Arthritis Rheum. **13:** 846, 1970.
6. Talbott, J.U.: Medicine, **38:** 173, 1959.
7. Paik, C.H., Alavi, J., Dunea, G. and Weiner, L.: J.A.M.A. **213:** 296, 1970.

Author's address:

Prof. Dr. O. Sperling
Beilinson Medical Center
Dept. Clinical Biochemistry
Petah-Tikva
Israel

Fortschritte der Urol. und Nephrol. **16**, 36–42 (1981)
Steinkopff Verlag Darmstadt

Renal Excretion of Urate in Mammals

Françoise Roch-Ramel and Christian Schäli

Institut de Pharmacologie de l'Université de Lausanne, Lausanne, Switzerland.

Introduction

In almost all mammals the end product of purine metabolism is allantoin. Only in man and the great apes who have phylogenetically lost uricase activity, is uric acid the main product of purine metabolism. The absence of uricase is responsible for the high concentration of urate in human plasma as compared to lower mammals, and compels the kidneys to play a major role in the elimination of uric acid (Florkin and Duchateau, 1943). Defects in the renal excretory mechanisms, therefore, may induce disease in man by causing hyperuricemia. Lower mammalian species are not subject to hyperuricemia, the liver being the main organ for eliminating uric acid by converting it into allantoin.
Even though the physiological role of the kidney in eliminating urate in lower mammals is minor, it has been shown that there are no major differences in the mechanisms by which kidneys of different mammalian species transport urate (Roch-Ramel and Peters, 1978, review).

Urate excretion in man

Man excretes urate very inefficiently. The major fraction of the plasma urate is not protein bound and is freely filtrable (Steele, 1978, review). However 90% of the filtrable amount is transported back to the plasma by the reabsorptive mechanism ($D_{urate} <$ GFR) This reabsorptive transport is counteracted by a secretory mechanism which in particular conditions has been found to be more important than the reabsorption, leading to net secretion of urate ($C_{urate} >$GFR) (Steele, 1978). There is at present no doubt about the simultaneous occurence of reabsorption and secretion in man, as proposed by Gutman and Yü in their "Three component hypothesis" involving the filtration, secretion, and reabsorption of urate (Gutman and Yü, 1961).
Attemps have been made to evaluate the impotance of the secretory transport of urate in man by using pharmacologic agents. A "pyrazinamide suppression test" was developed by Steele and Rieselbach (1967).
Pyrazinamide is an antituberculosus drug which may induce hyperuricemia. The active substance, in fact, is pyrazinoic acid, a metabolite of pyrazinamide (Weiner and Tinker, 1972). When a large dose of pyrazinamide (3g) is administered to man, the concentration of pyrazinoic acid in the plasma reaches 10 to 20 mg/liter (Prasad et al., 1977), and the urinary excretion of urate falls to 20% of its control value, the fractional excretion of urate (FE_{urate}) to 2–3% (Steele, 1978). The "PZA suppressible excretion of urate" represents only a fraction of the total secretion because it does not comprise the part of secreted urate which is reabsorbed. Only if the secretory transport were located below

the reabsorptive transport, would the "pyrazinamide suppression test" measure total secretion (Steele 1978). As will be discussed below the reabsorptive transport, however, opposed to the secretory transport in the same tubular segments. It may be argued that the decrease of urate excretion induced by pyrazinoic acid reflects stimulation of the reabsorptive mechanism, rather than inhibition of the secretory mechanism. A few arguments, are against the assumption of a stimulation of the reabsorptive transport. Thus in the rat, pyrazinamide inhibits the reabsorptive transport of urate studied by the tubular microinjection method (Kramp et al., 1971). Furthermore in Cebus monkeys treated with 2-nitro probenecid in order to inhibit the reabsorption of urate, the administration of pyrazinoic acid induces a decrease in the fractional delivery of urate to the late proximal tubule reflecting an inhibition of the secretory transport (Roch-Ramel and Weiner, 1975). Of more interest for man is the observation that in the chimpanzee, a species close to man, the dose response curve relating the concentration of pyrazinoic acid in the plasma to the fractional excretion of urate shows that at low concentrations of pyrazinoic acid in the plasma (10 mg/Liter) the fractional excretion of urate is decreased, the secretory flux being inhibited. At much higher concentrations (500 mg/Liter) the reabsorptive flux also becomes inhibited and the FE_{urate} increases and becomes lager than normal. (Fanelli and Weiner, 1973).

Is the secretory transport in man and chimpanzee quantitatively important? The fact that in the chimpanzee, which normally excretes 10% of the amount filtered, it is possible to increase the fractional excretion to 150% by mersalyl (a mercurial diuretic) points to an important secretory capacity (Fanelli et al., 1973). In man, secretion, is required for maintaining urate homeostasis since patients treated with pyrazinamide for tuberculosis may develop hyperuricemia (Emmerson, 1978 review). Furthermore, a retention of urate is observed when diuretics are given over long periods. Part of the retention is secondary to volume depletion and a stimulation of reabsorption (Steele, 1978), but at least in the case of thiazides a direct inhibition of the secretory transport cannot be excluded (Emmerson 1978, review). Such an effect was shown to occur in the rat (Weinman et al. 1975, 1976).

Tubular sites of urate transport, animal studies

The question, which parts of the nephron are responsible for the secretion or the reabsorption of urate cannot be easily solved by studies in man. Techniques giving direct access to renal tubules, such as tubular micropuncture and microperfusion (in vivo) (Lang et al., 1978) or microperfusion of isolated tubules (in vitro) (Chonko et al 1975) are needed. Wheras the micropuncture method cannot be used in man for ethical reasons, in vitro microperfusion may be used: however the dissection of tubules from pieces of human kidneys is difficult and kidneys are rarely available.

The technique of free flow micropuncture consists in the collection of fluid from different sites of the nephron. For urate, only data from superficial nephrons are available. The proximal and distal convoluted tubules of these nephrons reach the surface of the cortex. The pars recta of proximal tubules is not accessible. Progress in the micropuncture field was slow because a very sensitive method for the determination of urate was needed, the volume of tubular fluid collected being small (0.1 μliter) and the plasma urate concentration being low (table 1). Furthermore, all mammalian species have uricase activity

Table 1: Concentration of urate in the plasma (P_{urate}) and fractional excretion of urate (FE_{urate}) in mammals

	P_{urate} µm/l	mg %	FE_{urate}
man	300–400	5–6	0.10
rat	30– 60	0.5–1	0.20–0.4
mongrel dog	30– 60	0.5–1	0.30–0.4
cebus monkey	120–180	2 –3	0.05
rabbit	10– 20	0.3	0.6 –1.2
dalmatian dog	60–120	1 –2	0.8 –1.2
pig	3	0.05	2.0

which converts urate into allantoin and thus lowers the concentration of urate in the plasma. Several chemical or radiochemical analytical methods were used in micropuncture studies in the rat and discrepancies resulted from a lack of specificity or sensitivity of the methods used (Roch-Ramel and Peters, 1978). At present a specific and sensitive method based on HPLC amperometry is available (Pachla and Kissinger, 1975).
Free flow micropuncture experiments were performed in rats (Roch-Ramel et al., 1979–1980), dogs (Roch-Ramel et al., 1976a), Cebus monkeys (Roch-Ramel et al., 1980a), rabbits (Roch-Ramel et al., 1976b), and pigs (Roch-Ramel et al., 1980b). In table 2, the fractional deliveries of urate to different sites of the nephron and to the pelvic urine (FE_{urate}) are compared. In the three species excreting only a fraction of the filtered load, the rat, the mongrel dog, and the Cebus monkey net reabsorption was observed to occur along the proximal tubule: fractions equivalent to 36%, 50%, and 7% of the filtered load respectively reached the distal tubule.

Table 2: Comparison of fractional deliveries of urate.

	fractional deliveries of urate proximal tubule early	late	distal tubule	pelvic urine
rat	0.8	0.5	0.36	0.34
mongrel dog	0.7	0.5	0.50	0.47
cebus monkey	0.7	0.2	0.07	0.03
rabbit	0.8	0.8	– –	1.6
dalmatian dog	1.0	1.0	1.4	1.4
pig	4	4 –	– –	2.0

In the rabbit reabsorption occurred along the convoluted part, but net secretion along the pars recta of the proximal tubules (as proved by in vitro studies, Chonko et al., 1975, Schäli and Roch-Ramel, 1980a). In the Dalmatian dog, a strain of dog which has a genetic defect in urate transport, no net movement of urate occurred in the proximal convoluted tubule; and in the rabbit net secretion occurred into the pars recta (Roch-Ramel et al., 1976a). In the third species observed to secrete urate, the pig, in contrast, the convoluted part of the proximal tubule is a site of net secretion, whereas net reabsorption occurs in the pars recta so that the delivery of urate which was four times larger than the filtered load in the late proximal tubule, is only twice the filtered load when the urine reaches the pelvis (Roch-Ramel et al., 1980b).

In the rat, the Cebus monkey, and the mongrel dog it was shown that, along the proximal convoluted tubule, the reabsorptive movement is opposed by a secretory transport. In the dog (Roch-Ramel et al., 1976a) and in the Cebus monkey (Roch-Ramel and Weiner, 1975) the evidence is indirect, based on the decrease of urate delivery when pyrazinoic acid is given.

Direct evidence exists, however, for the rat proximal convoluted tubule to which the technique of continuous microperfusion has been applied. In this type of experiments the efflux or influx of urate out or into the tubular lumen is measured (Lang et al., 1972, Roch-Ramel and Peters, 1978, review).

In the rat both fluxes appear to have a large transporting capacity: the reabsorptive flux was not saturated when the concentration of urate in the lumen reached 1 mMol (Weinman et al., 1976) and the secretory flux became saturated only at a concentration of 1.3 mMol in the plasma (Weinman et al., 1980).

Mechanisms involved in the tubular transports

The mechanisms involved in urate reabsorption are not well known. The reabsorptive mechanism in at least a few species represents "active transport": urate may be reabsorbed from tubular fluid of the Cebus monkey when the concentration of urate is smaller than in the plasma and smaller than that predicted by the transepithelial electrical potential difference at equilibrium. Furthermore, in man and the chimpanzee, the concentration of urate in urine becomes smaller than that in the plasma when the secretion of urate is inhibited by the administration of pyrazinoic or pyrazinamide (Roch-Ramel and Weiner, 1980, review).

In the rat, micropuncture studies showed that there is no direct coupling between sodium and urate reabsorption (Weinman et al., 1976). However, changes in extracellular volume influence urate reabsorption: dehydration increases it, whereas expansion of the extracellular volume depresses it, in the rat as well as in man (Steele 1978, or Emmerson, 1978, reviews).

Little is known about the specificity of the reabsorptive mechanism. Data from Knight et al. (1980) suggest that glucose and phloridizin may inhibit urate reabsorption. Urate and glucose might thus share the same transport mechanism. A large number of drugs inhibit the reabsorptive mechanism. Besides the well-known uricosuric drugs such as probenecid,sulfinpyrazone, and benziodarone, many other agents such as pyrazinamide, PAH or salicylate inhibit the reabsorptive mechanism in mammals (Roch-Ramel and Peters, 1978). That PZA also inhibits the reabsorption of urate in the chimpanzee has been demonstrated by Fanelli and Weiner (1973).

The fact that these drugs inhibit urate reabsorption does not imply that the FE of urate will increase: the excretion of urate depends on the relative drug sensitivity of the secretory mechanism versus that of the reabsorptive mechanism in different species. It is well known that probenecid is antiuricosuric in rabbits (Moller, 1966).

The specificity of the secretory mechanism appears to differ in different mammalian species. Endogenous substrates such as lactate or β-hydroxybutyrate are known to increase the blood urate concentration in man (Emmerson, 1978, review). This fact is generally interpreted as the consequence of an inhibition of the secretory mechanism. In lower mammals there are no clear-cut effects of these endogenous substrates (Roch-Ramel and Peters, 1978).

More is known about the competition of foreign substances, such as pra-aminohippurate (PAH) and pyrazinoic acid for urate transport. In man the excretion of urate is not decreased by the administration of PAH whereas pyrazinoic acid has a clear-cut effect (Boner and Steele, 1973, Steele and Rieselbach, 1967). In the Cebus monkey pyrazinoic acid also inhibits the secretion of urate, whereas PAH does not. The same is true for the rat. In other species, such as the pig and the rabbit, PAH is a good inhibitor of secretion whereas pyrazinoic acid is not (Simmonds et al., 1976, Schäli and Roch-Ramel, 1980b). Thus the systems involved in urate excretion do not appear to be identical in all mammalian species (Weiner, 1979, Roch-Ramel and Weiner, 1980, for review).

Conclusions

Renal transports of urate in the mammalian kidney have a common characteristic feature: a secretory and a reabsorptive transport oppose each other in the proximal tubule. The proximal tubule (pars convoluta and pars recta) plays the major role in urate transport. The secretory and the reabsorptive transports may be inhibited by the same drugs, the concentrations needed to inhibit one or the other differing in the different species. The secretory transport of urate may involve different carriers in different species. Further studies are needed to determine the role of the peritubular site versus the luminal site of the cells in the reabsorptive and the secretory transports and to characterize the carriers involved.

References

Boner, G., T.H. Steele: Relationship of urate and p-aminohippurate secretion in man. Am. J. Physiol. **225** 100–104 (1973).

Chonko, A.M., C.M. Lowe, J.J. Grantham: Uric acid secretion in isolated perfused rabbit kidney tubules: comparison of proximal convoluted, proximal straight and cortical collecting segments. Clin. Res. **23:** abstr. 538A (1975).

Emmerson, B.T.: Abnormal urate excretion associated with renal and systemic disorders, drugs, and toxins. In: W.N. Kelley, I.M. Weiner (eds.). Handbook of Experimental Pharmacology, Vol. **51:** Uric Acid. Berlin: Springer, 1978, p. 287–324.

Fanelli, G.M., Jr., I.M. Weiner: Pyrazinoate excretion in the chimpanzee: relation to urate disposition and the actions of uricosuric drugs. J. Clin. Invest. **52:** 1946–1957 (1973).

Fanelli, G.M., Jr., D.L. Bohn, S.S. Reilly, I.M. Weiner: Effects of mercurial diuretics on renal transport of urate in the chimpanzee. Am. J. Physiol. **224:** 985–992 (1973).

Florkin, M., G. Duchateau: Les formes du système enzymatique de l'uricolyse et l'évolution du catabolisme purique chez les animaux. Arch. Int. Physiol. **53:** 267–307 (1943).

Gutman, A.B., T.F. Yu: A three-component system for regulation of renal excretion of uric acid in man. Trans. Assoc. Am. Physicians **74:** 353–364 (1961).

Knight, T.F., H.O. Senekjian, S.C. Sansom, E.J. Weinman: Proximal tubule glucose efflux in the rat as a function of delivered load. Am. J. Physiol. **238:** (Renal Fluid Electrolyte Physiol. 7): F499–F503 (1980).

Kramp, R.A., W.E. Lassiter, C.W. Gottschalk: Urate-2-^{14}C transport in the rat nephron. J. Clin. Invest. **50** 35–48 (1971).
Lang, F., R. Greger, P. Deetjen: Handling of uric acid by the rat kidney. II. Microperfusion studies on bidirectional transport of uric acid in the proximal tubule. Pfluegers Arch. **335:** 257–265 (1972).
Lang, F., R. Greger, C. Lechene, F.G. Knox: Micropuncture techniques. In: M. Martinez-Maldonado (ed.). Methods in Pharmacology, Vol. **48:** Renal Pharmacology. New York, London: Plenum Press 1978, p. 75–103.
Møller, J.V.: Clearance experiments on the effect of probenecid on urate excretion in the rabbit. Acta Pharmacol. Toxicol. (Kbh.) **23:** 321–328 (1966).
Pachla, L.A., P.T. Kissinger: Estimation of serum uric acid by high performance liquid chromatography with electrochemical detection. Clin. Chim. Acta **59:** 309–312 (1975).
Prasad, D.R., I.M. Weiner, T.H. Steele: Diuretic-induced uricosuria: interaction with pyrazinoate transport in man. J. Pharmacol. Exp. Ther. **200:** 58–64 (1977).
Roch-Ramel, F., G. Peters: Urinary excretion of uric acid in nonhuman mammalian species. In: W.N. Kelley, I.M. Weiner (eds.). Handbook of Experimental Pharmacology, Vol. **51:** Uric Acid. Berlin: Springer, 1978, p. 211–255.
Roch-Ramel, F., I.M. Weiner: Inhibition of urate excretion by pyrazinoate: a micropuncture study. Am. J. Physiol. **229:** 1604–1608 (1975).
Roch-Ramel, F., I.M. Weiner: Renal excretion of urate: factors determining the actions of drugs. Kidney Int. **18:** 665–676 (1980).
Roch-Ramel, F., N.L.M. Wong, J.H. Dirks: Renal excretion of urate in mongrel and Dalmatian dogs: a micropuncture study. Am. J. Physiol. **231:** 326–331 (1976a).
Roch-Ramel, F., D. de Rougemont, G. Peters, I.M. Weiner: Micropuncture study of urate excretion by the kidney of the rat, the Cebus monkey and the rabbit. In: S. Silbernagl, F. Lang, R. Greger (eds.). Amino Acid Transport and Uric Acid Transport. Symposium Innsbruck, June 1975. Stuttgart: Thieme, 1976b, p. 188–192.
Roch-Ramel, F., F. Granges, L. Roth, J. Widmer, I.M. Weiner: Renal handling of urate by nondiuretic and diuretic rats: HPLC-amperometric determination of urate concentrations. Renal Physiol. **2:** 122–129 (1979/80).
Roch-Ramel, F., D. Diezi-Chomety, L. Roth, I.M. Weiner: A micropuncture study of urate excretion by *Cebus* monkeys employing high performance liquid chromatography with amperometric detection of urate. Pfluegers Arch. **383:** 203–207 (1980a).
Roch-Ramel, F., F. White, L. Vowles, H.A. Simmonds, J.S. Cameron: Micropuncture study of tubular transport of urate and PAH in the pig kidney. Am. J. Physiol. **239:** (Renal Fluid Electrolyte Physiol. 8): F107–F112 (1980b).
Schäli, Ch., F. Roch-Ramel: Accumulation of [^{14}C]urate and [^{3}H]PAH in isolated proximal tubular segments of the rabbit kidney. Am J. Physiol. **239:** (Renal Fluid Electrolyte Physiol. 8): F222–F227 (1980a).
Schali, Ch., F. Roch-Ramel: Transport of urate and para-aminohippurate in isolated, nonperfused proximal renal tubules of the pig kidney. Kidney Int. **17:** 860–861 (1980b) (abstr.).
Simmonds, H.A., P.J. Hatfield, J.S. Cameron, A. Cadenhead: Uric acid excretion by the pig kidney. Am. J. Physiol. **230:** 1654–1661 (1976).
Steele, T.H. Urate excretion in man, normal and gouty. In: W.N. Kelley, I.M. Weiner (eds.) Handbook of Experimental Pharmacology, Vol **51:** Uric Acid. Berlin: Springer, 1978, p. 257–286.
Steele, T.H., R.E. Rieselbach: The renal mechanism for urate homeostasis in normal man. Am. J. Med. **43:** 868–875 (1967).
Weiner, I.M.: Urate transport in the nephron. Am. J. Physiol. **237:** (Renal Fluid Electrolyte Physiol. 6): F85–F92 (1979).
Weiner, I.M., J.P. Tinker: Pharmacology of pyrazinamide: metabolic and renal function studies related to the mechanism of drug-induced urate retention J Pharmacol. Exp. Ther. **180:** 411–434 (1972).
Weinman, E.J., G. Eknoyan, W.N. Suki: The influence of the extracellular fluid volume on the tubular reabsorption of uric acid. J. Clin. Invest. **55:** 283–291 (1975).
Weinman, E.J., D. Steplock, W.N. Suki, G. Eknoyan: Urate reabsorption in proximal convoluted tubule of the rat kidney. Am. J. Physiol. **231:** 509–515 (1976).

Weinman, E.J., S.C. Sansom, D.A. Steplock, A.U. Sheth, T.F. Knight, H.O. Senekjian: Secretion of urate in the proximal convoluted tubule of the rat. Am. J. Physiol. **239:** (Renal Fluid Electrolyte Physiol. 8): F383–F387 (1980).

Author's address:

Dr. *F Roch-Ramel*
Institut de Pharmacologie
Universite de Lausanne
Lausanne
Switzerland

Fortschritte der Urol. und Nephrol. **16**, 43–47 (1981)
Steinkopff Verlag Darmstadt

Relation Between Urate Transport and Tubular Flow Rate in Rat and Man

P. Deetjen, F. Lang, and R. Greger

Institute of Physiology, University of Innsbruck, Innsbruck, Austria

Fractional excretion of urate in man follows a distinct circadian rhythm. This rhythm is monophasic and normally parallels that of urine flow rate (Fig. 1). However, if urine flow rate is enhanced by excessive drinking of tap water, there is no concomittant increase of urate excretion (6). On the other hand, if osmotic diuresis is induced by the infusion of mannitol, uric acid excretion increases significantly (Fig. 2).

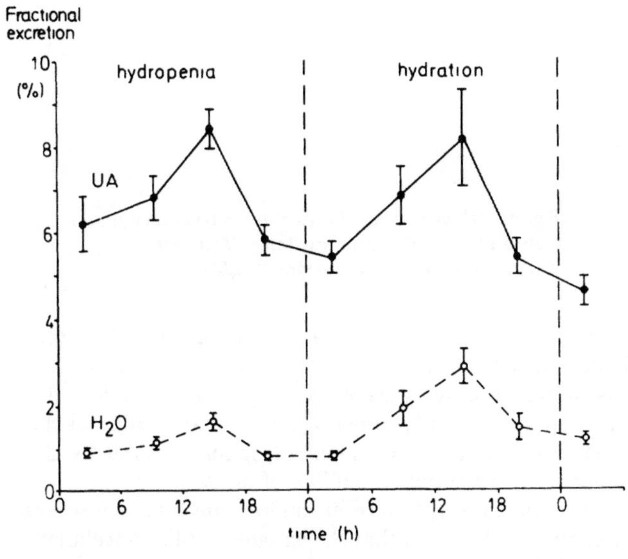

Fig. 1: Fractional excretion of uric acid (closed symbols) and water (open symbols) in man: diurnal variation during hydropenia (left) and during water diuresis (right). All values are means ±SEM.

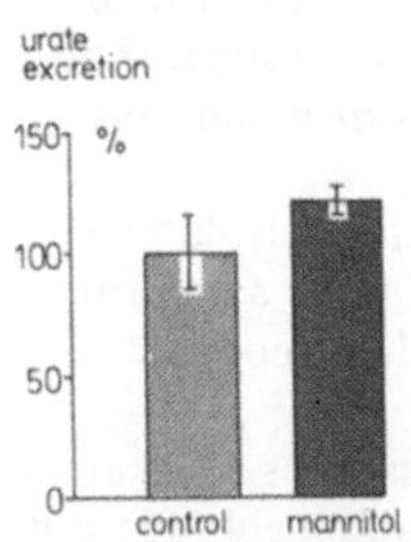

Fig. 2: Effect of mannitol on fractional excretion of urate in man (means ± SEM, significantly different [$p < 0.05$] at paired comparison).

This discrepancy is easily explained by results of previous studies which we have performed in rats using microperfusion techniques in single nephron segments. From these experiments it is apparent (Fig. 3) that fractional urate reabsorption in the loop of Henle dramatically decreases when intraluminal flow rate increases. At physiological flow rates of 10 nl/min urate reabsorption is 3 times higher than at a perfusion rate of 40 nl/min (2). Meanwhile our findings have been extended by Senekjian et al. (8), who demonstrated that also in the convoluted part of the proximal tubule urate reabsorption decreases with luminal flow rate.

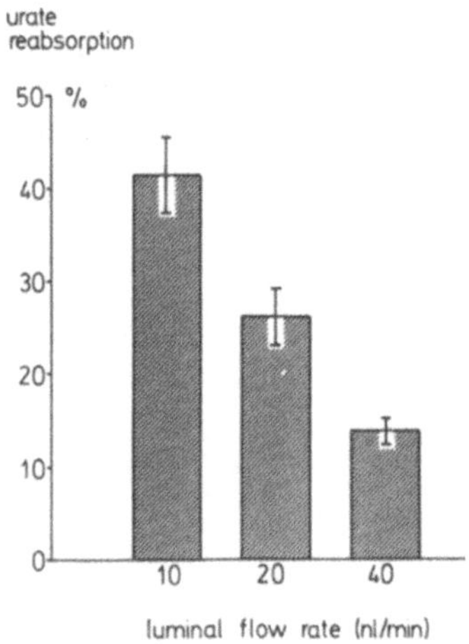

Fig. 3: Effect of liminal flow rate on fractional urate reabsorption in the loops of Henle. Microperfusion studies in the rat (means ± SEM).

This dependency of urate reabsorption on intratubular flow velocity suggests that contact time along the urate permeable part of the nephron is the main determinant of urate reabsorption. Urate permeability, however, only exists along the proximal tubule including Henle's loop while the distal nephron is nearly impermeable to urate. Thus, all changes in intratubular flow rate during water diuresis which take place solely in the distal nephron have no significant influence on the tubular handling of urate.
The proximal flow dependency of urate reabsorption offers an interpretation for several unexplained findings: It is well known (1, 5, 8, 12) that the expansion of extracellular volume leads to uricosuria. Volume expansion, however, may increase glomerular tration rate (GFR) and it reduces sodium chloride and water reabsorption in the proximal tubule. Both effects result in an augmentation of intratubular flow rate. Since the proximal tubule has a limited distensibility, linear flow velocity is accelerated and contact time inversely shortened. This in turn limits urate reabsorption and leads to uricosuria. If during volume expansion intratubular flow rate is kept constant by experimental means—as Senekjian et al. have shown (8)—then no uricosuric effect occurs.
In general, all diuretic maneuvers which acutely enhance flow rate in the convoluted and/or straight proximal tubule may produce uricosuria (5). In contrast, chronic administration especially of high-ceiling diuretics which produce extracellular volume contraction results in antiuricosuria (5, 8, 11).
In the course of renal insufficiency a loss of nephrons develops. This imposes a higher excretory load on the remaining nephrons. To balance extracellular sodium chloride and

fluid, these nephrons have to cut down isotonic fluid reabsorption in the proximal nephron. This, however, enhances luminal flow rate. A reduced urate reabsorption is expected. Fig. 4 demonstrates that fractional urate excretion is indeed increased in advanced renal failure.

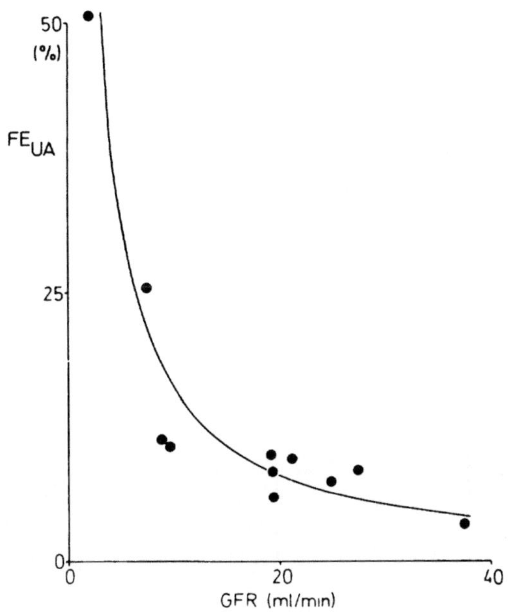

Fig. 4: Fractional urate excretion (FE_{UA}) as a function of glomerular filtration rate (GFR) in patients with renal insufficiency.

The observation that the suppressive effect of pyrazinamide is more marked in renal insufficiency has led to the speculation that stimulation of urate secretion accounts for a relative uricosuria in renal insufficiency (9). However, a more simple explanation is that reduced reabsorption of secreted urate will enhance the excretion of secreted urate and will yield increased sensitivity to pyrazinamide as well as increased secretion per se.
Glucose has been reported to inhibit urate transport, presumably by enhancing intracellular sodium concentration (3). Apart from this effect glucose may be expected to influence urate reabsorption by modulating luminal flow rate: Glucose transport in the proximal nephron is coupled to sodium transport in the proximal nephron. Thus, the presence of glucose stimulates isotonic fluid reabsorption in that nephron segment. Fig. 5 demonstrates that glucose loading may indeed reduce fractional excretion of urate. It must be pointed out that enhancement of the filtered glucose load beyond the maximal threshold concentration may lead to the opposite effect, since nonreabsorbed glucose reduces volume reabsorption by osmotic forces.
Altered isotonic fluid reabsorption in the proximal nephron mediates variations of fractional urate excretion during circadian rhythm, diuretic treatment, renal insufficiency,

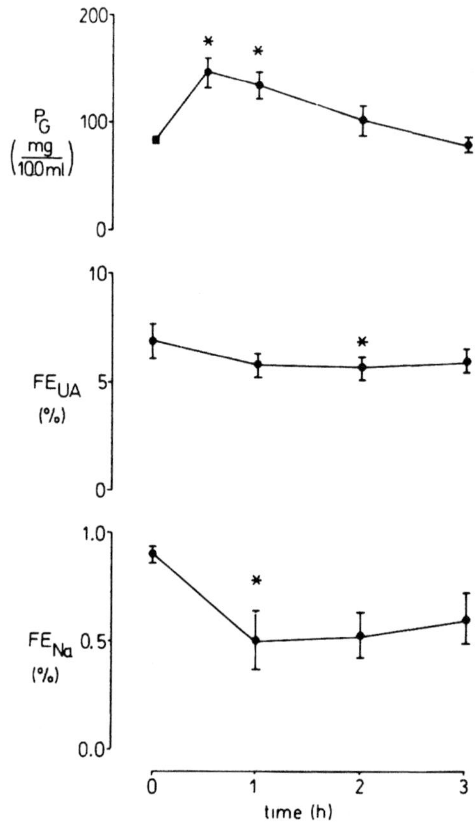

Fig. 5: Fractional excretion of urate (FE_{UA}) and of sodium (FE_{Na}) in man following enhancement of plasma glucose levels (PG) by an oral glucose load (means ± SEM, * = significantly different [$p < 0.05$] from control value at paired comparison).

and hyperglycemia. It is tempting to speculate that the dependency of urate reabsorption on flow rate in the proximal nephron also accounts for, or at least contributes to, altered urate excretion in a number of other experimental conditions and clinical situations, such as metabolic alkalosis, Fanconi's syndrome, cystinosis, heavy metal poisoning, sickle cell anemia, Wilson's disease, acute renal failure, renal transplants, and unilateral nephrectomy.

Up to now we have no definite proof for this hypothesis. However, the contribution of altered luminal flow rate to antiuricosuria or uricosuria in a variety of clinical situations seems to be a plausible interpretation.

References

1. Greger, R., Lang, F., and Deetjen, P.: Handling of uric acid by the rat kidney. I. Microanalysis of uric acid in proximal tubular fluid. Pflügers Arch. **324:** 279, 1971.

2. Greger, R., Lang, F., and Deetjen, P.: Urate handling by the rat kidney. IV. Reabsorption in the loops of Henle. Pflügers Arch. **352:** 115, 1974.
3. Knight, T.F., Senekjian, H.O., Sansom, S., Weinman, E.J.: Effects of intraluminal D-glucose and probenecid on urate absorption in the rat procimal tubule. Am. J. Physiol. **236:** F526–F529, 1979.
4. Lang, F.: Parameters and Mechanisms of urate transport in the rat kidney. Internat. Symp. on amino acid transport and uric acid transport (Eds. S. Silbernagl, F. Lang, R. Greger) Georg Thieme Verlag, Stuttgart (1975).
5. Lang, F., Greger, R. and Deetjen, P.: Effect of Diuretics on Uric Acid Metabolism and Excretion. In: Diuretics in Research and Clinics (Eds.: W. Siegenthaler, R. Beckerhoff, W. Vetter) Georg Thieme Verlag, Stuttgart (1977).
6. Lang, F., Greger, R., Oberleithner, H., Griss, E., Lang, K., Pastner, D., Dittrich, P. and Deetjen, P.: Renal handling of urate in healthy man in hyperuricaemia and renal insufficiency: circadian fluctuation, effect of water diuresis and of uricosuric agents. Europ. J. Clin. Invest. **10:** 285–291, 1980.
7. Oelert, H., Baumann, K., and Gekle, D.: Permeabilitatsmessungen einiger schwacher organischer Säuren aus dem distalen Konvolut der Rattenniere. Pflügers Arch. **307:** 178, 1969.
8. Senekjian, H.O., Knight, T.F., Sansom, S.C., and Weinman, E.J.: Effect of flow rate and the extracellular fluid volume on proximal urate and water absorption. Kidney Int. **17:** 155–161, 1980.
9. Steele, T.H. and Rieselbach, R.E.: The renal mechanism for urate homeostasis in normal man. The contribution of residual nephrons within the chronically diseased kidney to urate homeostasis in man. Am. J. Med. **43:** 868, 1967.
10. Steele, T.H. and Oppenheimer, S.: Factors affecting urate excretion following diuretic administration in man. Am. J. Med. **47:** 564, 1969.
11. Steele, T.H. Urate excretion in man, normal and gouty. In: Handbook of experimental pharmacology **51:** (1978)
12 Weinman, E.J., Eknoyan, G., and Suki, W.N.: The influence of the extracellular fluid volume on the tubular reabsorption of uric acid. J. Clin. Invest. **55:** 283, 1975.

Author's address:

Prof. Dr. *P. Deetjen*
Institut für Physiologie der
Universitat Innsbruck
6010 Innsbruck
Austria

Fortschritte der Urol. und Nephrol. 16, 48–51 (1981)
Steinkopff Verlag Darmstadt

Renal Tubular Handling of Urate in Calcium Stone Formers with Hyperuricosuria or Renal Acidification Defects

B. Fellström, U. Backman, B. G. Danielson, G. Johansson, S. Ljunghall, and B. Wikström

Department of Internal Medicine, University Hospital, Uppsala, Sweden

Introduction

Hyperuricosuria has been considered as a risk factor for calcium stone formation (1) and thought to be mainly a result of consumption of purine rich animal protein (2). According to Coe (3) some hyperuricosuric patients could not decrease their excretion of urate on a low purine diet to the same extent as controls and he suggested that a defect in the renal handling of urate may exist. We have earlier shown (4) that stone formers with a proximal renal tubular acidosis (pRTA) have a higher serum urate than patients with a normal acidification of the urine. Hyperuricemic patients with RTA also have a lower urate excretion than hyperuri cemic patients with a normal acidification of the urine (4). The aim of the present study was to investigate if hyperuricosuria or renal acidification defects in calcium stone disease were associated with a dysfunction in the renal tubular handling of urate. Furthermore, the object was to find out to what extent serum and urinary urate could be explained in terms of renal tubular transport phenomena.

Material and Methods

A total of 28 recurrent calcium stone patients and 12 healthy controls were studied. Twelve patients had hyperuricosuria (urinary urate $>$ 4.5 mmol/24h in males and $>$ 4.0 mmol/24h in females, which was mean ± S D in healthy controls), eight patients had a proximal (pRTA), and eight had a distal (dRTA) renal tubular acidosis of the incomplete type. The patients, 23 males and five females, were referred from our outpatient stone clinic and the controls, eight males and four females, were recruited from the staff. The subjects were studied after an overnight's fasting and asked to drink 300–400 ml of water in the morning to increase diuresis. After urine collections during two 30-minute periods, 3g pyrazinamide (PZA) were given orally to suppress the tubular secretion of urate. After 90 minutes another three consecutive 30-min urine collections were made. Venous samples for urate and creatinine analysis were drawn in the middle of the urine collection periods.

Glomerular filtration rate (GFR) was estimated through endogenous creatinine clearance and the rate of urate filtration from GFR and serum urate. The pyrazinamide suppressible part of the urate excretion was the intial excretion (UV-ur) minus the minimum excretion during PZA suppression (UV-ur, min). The tubular reabsorption of filtered urate (TR-ur) was calculated from GFR and the minimum urate clearance during PZA suppression. The amount of filtered urate not being reabsorbed was calculated from the filtered and reabsorbed urate (5).

Serum and the 24-hour urinary excretion of urate under nonfasting conditions had been measured in advance. Renal acidification defects were diagnosed through a short ammonium chloride load (6).

Results

There was no difference in glomerular filtration rate between stone formers and controls or between the subgroups of stone formers (Table 1). Hyperuricosuric patients had a slightly higher serum urate than the others. The pre-pyrazinamide excretion of urate was equal in all groups except in patients with dRTA who had a lower excretion than the others. Correspondingly the PZA-suppressible fraction of the urate excretion was lower in patients with dRTA than in the others. During pyrazinamide the excretion was suppressed in all subjects to 3–31% of the basal excretion. In patients with pRTA the suppression was more pronounced than in controls and also occured earlier in time. The tubular reabsorption of filtered urate was in the range of 98.4–99.8% and was significantly higher in patients with pRTA than in both controls and patients with hyperuricosuria (Table 1).

Table 1: Pre- and postpyrazinamide urate data in stone formers and controls (mean ±1 SD in groups).

	Controls	Hyperuricosuria	pRTA	dRTA
Number of subjects	12	12	8	8
S-urate (μmol/l)	304 ± 51	373 ± 72[a]	302 ± 50	347 ± 102
GFR (ml/min)	129 ± 27	131 ± 35	125 ± 22	112 ± 51
UV-urate (μmol/min)	2.7 ± 0.9	2.9 ± 1.0	2.9 ± 1.0	1.9 ± 0.8[b]
UV-urate, min (μmol/min)	0.31 ± 0.14	0.33 ± 0.18	0.21 ± 0.06	0.26 ± 0.15
$\frac{\text{UV-urate, min}}{\text{UV-urate}}$ (%)	12 ± 4	12 ± 6	8 ± 4[c]	14 ± 9
TR-urate (%)	99.2 ± 0.2	99.1 ± 0.3	99.4 ± 0.1[d]	99.1 ± 0.5

[a] $p < 0.02$ compared to controls or pRTA
[b] $p < 0.05$ compared to hyperuricosuria or pRTA
[b] $p < 0.05$ compared to hyperuricosuria
[d] $p < 0.02$ compared to controls and $p < 0.01$ compared to hyperuricosuria

pRTA = proximal renal tubular acidification defect
dRTA = distal tubular renal acidification defect
UV-urate = excretion of urate
TR-urate = tubular reabsorptional filtred urate

There was no correlation between fasting or nonfasting serum urate on the one hand and basal urate excretion or the PZA-suppressible fraction of urate excretion on the other hand. Neither was there any correlation between the 24-hour urate excretion and the fasting excretion.

The tubular reabsorption of urate was positively correlated to the nonfasting serum urate ($p < 0.05$) and inversely correlated to the 24-hour excretion of urate ($p < 0.01$). The amount of nonreabsorbed filtered urate extrapolated to 24 hours was in the range 0.05–1.16 mmol/24h. The amount of urinary urate calculated this way was positively correlated to the measured 24-hour urinary excretion of urate ($r = 0.55$, $p < 0.001$) and accounted for up to 24% of the 24-hour excretion.

Discussion

In the normal human kidney 98–100% of the filtered urate is reabsorbed. Substrate regulated secretion and postsecretory reabsorption of urate are considered to be the quantitatively most important renal transport systems for the regulation of the urinary excretion of urate (7).
All the hyperuricosuric patients in this investigation had a urate clearance of the same order as the controls. Only one hyperuricosuric patient had a clearance urate/clearance creatinine of 14.5%, thus exceeding the 95% tolerance limit in the controls. In this patient, however, 95% of the excretion was PZA suppressible. The PZA-suppressible fraction of urate excretion and the tubular reabsorption of filtered urate in hyperuricosuric stone formers did not differ from the controls. Thus it is concluded that the renal tubular handling of urate in hyperuricosuric calcium stone patients does not differ from that of healthy subjects.
Patients with a proximal renal tubular acidification defect had a basal urate excretion not different from controls or hyperuricosuric patients. Their response to pyrazinamide was, however, more pronounced than in controls and hyperuricosuric patients. The calculated tubular reabsorption of filtered urate was higher than in both controls and hyperuricosuric patients. It is suggested that this may contribute to the higher serum urate and the lower urate clearance in stone formers with a proximal renal acidification defect compared to patients with a normal acidification of the urine that we have reported on previously (4).
This view is supported by the fact that the tubular reabsorption of urate was positively correlated to the nonfasting serum urate and inversely correlated to the 24-hour urinary urate excretion. The quantitative importance of this seemingly small variation in the tubular reabsorption of filtered urate (98.4–99.8%) can be estimated by calculating the corresponding amount of urate during a 24-hour period. It could be shown that this amount of urinary urate is not only positively correlated to the measured 24-hour urinary excretion of urate ($p < 0.001$) but would also account for up to 24% of the 24-hour excretion. It is therefore suggested that the degree of reabsorption of filtered urate is important for both the serum and the urinary excretion of urate under normal nonfasting conditions.

References

1 Coe, F.L., Kavalach, A.G.: Hypercalciuria and hyperuricosuria in patients with calcium nephrolithiasis. New. Engl. J. Med. **291:** 1344–1350 (1974).

2 Robertson, W.G., Heyburn, P.J., Peacock, M., Hanes, F.A., Swaminathan, R.: The effects of high animal protein intake on the risk of calcium stone formation in the urinary tract. Clin. Sci. **57:** 285–288 (1979).

3. Coe, F.L. Nephrolithiasis. Pathogenesis and treatment. Year Book Medical Publishers 1978, pp 95- Chicago and London.
4. Fellström, B., Backman, U., Danielson, B.G., Johansson, G., Ljunghall, S., Wikström, B.: Urate metabolism and urinary acidification. Fourth International Symposium on Urolithiasis Research, Williamsburg 1980. In press.
5. Steele, T.H.: Urate excretion in man, normal and gouty. In: Uric acid, (Eds. W.N. Kelley & I.M. Weiner) Springer Verlag 1978, pp 257–286.
6. Backman, U., Danielson, B.G., Johansson, G., Ljunghall, S., Wikström, B.: Incidence and clinical importance of renal tubular defects in recurrent renal stone formers. Nephron **25:** 96–101 (1980).
7. Sorensen, L.B., Levinson, D.J.: Evidence for four compartments in the renal handling of uric acid in man. In: Amino Acid Transport and Uric Acid Transport. (Eds. S. Silbernagl, F. Lang, R. Greger) Georg Thieme Publishers, 1976, pp 243–247.

Author's address:

Dr. *B. Fellstrom*
Dept. of Internal Medicine
University Hospital
75014 Uppsala
Sweden

Fortschritte der Urol. und Nephrol. 16, 52–57 (1981)
Steinkopff Verlag Darmstadt

'Uric Acid' Stones in Children: Problems of Diagnosis and Treatment in a New Defect– Adenine Phosphoribosyltransferase Deficiency

H. A. Simmonds[1], J. S. Cameron[1], M. J. Dillon[2], T. M. Barratt[2], and K. J. Van Acker[3]

1 Clinical Science Laboratories, Guy's Hospital, London, S.E.1. U.K.
2 Hospital for Sick Children, Great Ormond Street, London, W.1., U.K.
3 Universitaire Instelling Antwerpen, Universiteitsplein 1, 2610 Wilrijk, Belgium

Uric acid stones generally represent less than 10% of all renal stones in most adult populations. Stones *per se* are rare in childhood. In some instances a metabolic basis in purine metabolism may be identified (Delete) as the cause of uric acid stones (1). This results

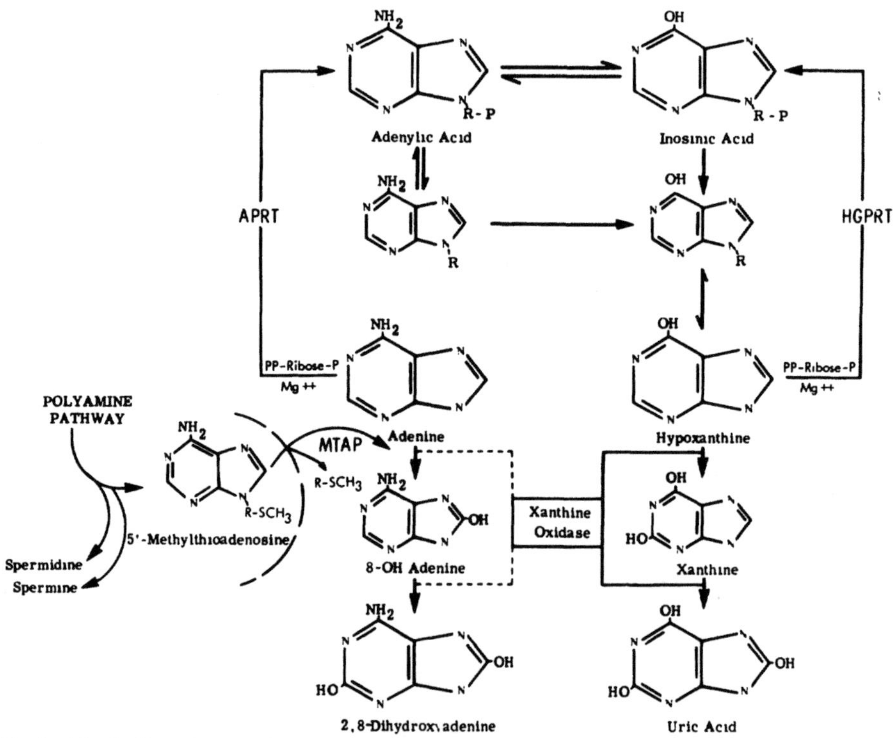

Fig. 1: Metabolic pathways of purine metabolism showing the role of the salvage enzymes HGPRT and APRT and the alternative route of adenine metabolism when APRT is absent of inhibited. Adenine is not a product of purine nucleotide degradation in man but is produced as a by-product of the polyamine pathway.

from a partial or complete deficiency of the enzyme hypoxanthine guanine phosphoribosyltransferase (HGPRT). In the latter (better known as the Lesch-Nyhan syndrome) gout, severe mental retardation, spasticity, self-mutilation and other manifestations may co-exist (1).

Recently a new cause of supposed 'uric acid' stones in children was identified independently by two groups (2, 3), a defect of the companion salvage enzyme adenine phosphoribosyltransferase (APRT). This results in an inability to salvage the purine base adenine, which is then picked up by xanthine oxidase and converted to the extremely insoluble analogue of uric acid, 2,8-dihydroxyadenine (2,8-DHA) (Fig. 1). In contrast to HGPRT deficiency, other than the urolithiasis, these children are normal and heterozygotes have no clinical abnormality.

In the short space of five years another nine cases (4–10) have been identified (Table 1), which would indicate that the defect is more prevalent than its recent description sug-

Table 1: Summary of published laboratory and clinical data in the nine homozygotes for APRT deficiency identified to date showing the extremes of clinical expression which may be encountered in this defect.

Patient	Year	Sex	Age* (yr.)	Original presentation	Onset (age)	Initially diagnosed by	APRT activity (nmol/mgHb/h) (Normal 24.5 ± 4.8)
London							
B.Dh. (3)	1975	M	$2\frac{1}{2}$	"Uric acid" stones	Birth	Adenine in urine	< 0.30
F.Dh. (4)	1976	M	7	Asymptomatic brother B.Dh.	Never ill	Family study	< 0.25
S.Rz. (5)	1977	F	19m	Stones (l. ureter, r. pelvis)	1 yr	2,8-DHA in stones	0.61
Sk.B. (6)	1979	F	4	Comatose, anuric Bilateral obstructive uropathy	2 yrs	Stones by ultrasound 2,8-DHA in stones	11.0** (1) < 0.01** (2)
Paris							
P.Tho. (2)	1974	M	$3\frac{1}{2}$	"Uric acid" stones	2 yrs	Negligible APRT activity in RBC's	< 0.002
L.B. (7)	1979	M	2	Stones (l. pelvis)	1 yr	2,8-DHA in stones (infra-red)	< 0.005
J.B. (8)	1979	F	14	Asymptomatic sister L.B.	Never ill	Family study	< .004
Innsbruck							
H.Er. (9)	1978	M	10	Acute renal failure "Uric acid" stones (Now on dialysis)	18 mths	2,8-DHA in urine stones not available	< .005
T.M. (10)	1980	M	6	"Uric acid" stone	6 yrs	2,8-DHA in stones (X-ray diffraction)	< .006

* at Delete correct diagnosis ** (1) packed cell transfusion on admission (2) 6 months later

The wide spectrum of clinical manifestation shown in the table would certainly o mask the true incidence. Two children have had no clinical manifestation and :ame to attention during the family study (4, 8). Two others have presented ıcute anuric renal failure, eventually pinpointed as being due to bilateral obstructive thy (6, 9). Both have suffered severe and permanent renal damage. One is now on a ic dialysis programme, the stones having been incorrectly identified (and treated) : acid over ten years (9).

ʼf the two most recent cases (described only in abstract) (11) from Japan is the first to be identified. Predictably here too there appears to have been serious deteriora- ı renal function (11), suggesting that renal, as well as stone clinics should be ıed for adults likely to be homozygotes for APRT deficiency and 2,8-DHA lithiasis.

ɜ seven stone formers described in detail, in six of them (2, 3, 5, 6, 9, 10), the stone riginally identified incorrectly, often repeatedly, as uric acid when analysed by con- ınal techniques (colorimetric or murexide test, thermogravimetric analysis). In one one was considered to be calcium oxalate (7). The reason for the repeated confusion -DHA with uric acid is the similarity in their chemical structure which causes them ct identically, mole for mole, in the above routine tests. The stones may be distin- :d in the laboratory only by the use of specialised techniques: UV spectrum in acid kali; infra red; mass spectrometry or x-ray crystallography. They are predominantly)8%) 2,8-DHA, with the remainder mostly uric acid (2, 3).

o correct stone identification, if specialist techniques are not availalble, include the rance of stones: 2,8-DHA are whitish to pale grey, rough, friable and crush with ɪric acid stones are yellowish, hard, smooth, round and crush with difficulty. Only :id will be acted on by uricase; the solubility of 2,8-DHA will not improve within ıysiological pH range; 2,8-DHA will separate in the acid, not the alkaline, fraction a technique of wet chemistry (6). Where possible, supposed uric acid stones should ısly be analysed by specific techniques.

ptomatic, non-stone-forming homozygotes may be identified by the adenine, as well 8-hydroxyadenine and 2,8-DHA excreted in the urine (generally in the approxi- proportion 1:0.3:1.5), or the absence of detectable APRT activity in lysed ery- ytes. These tests will also be essential to identify homozygotes where the stone is no · available (9), or not immediately identifiable as the cause of the clinical manifesta- 6). Here too problems may be encountered–APRT activity was falsely raised (Table .he erythrocytes of the child presenting with coma and acute renal failure because a d cell transfusion was necessary for anaemia on admission (6). Several months had pse before donor red cells (with normal activity) were eliminated from the circula- Table 1) and the lack of detectable APRT activity established (6).

: other case with severe renal damage the real cause of the original "uric acid" stone tion was eventually established from the identification of 2,8-DHA in the urine by ' (9). However, unless a special separation system is devised the 2,8-DHA will be ɜd by uric acid. It will also be undetectable if monitored only at 254 nm. Likewise a peak eluting in the adenine position, but really a methylated xanthine, may result in ·oneous diagnosis if the subject is not on a caffeine-free diet when studied (6).

ine has also been identified erroneously in the urine of a child with severe immu- ˈiciency due to another purine enzyme defect, adenosine deaminase (ADA) defi- y, as a result of degradation of deoxyadenosine in the cationic systems used (12). me levels as well as urine should thus be investigated.

There is a recurrent theme in the case reports of all affected patients–classic symptoms of urolithiasis in children, fever ascribed to urinary tract infection, macroscopic haematuria, dysuria, urinary retention and abdominal colics were present,in most instances within two years of birth, but were not always recognised as such (2–10). A lapse of up to two years generally occurred before the correct diagnosis of urolithiasis was made; from two to nine years (9) subsequently elapsed before the real stone component was identified and appropriate therapy instigated. Better knowledge of the disease and the use of more appropriate techniques is almost certainly responsible for the correct diagnosis being made almost as soon as the urolithiasis was recognised in the three most recent cases (5, 6, 10) (Table 1).

Treatment has also presented problems. One child was originally given allopurinol with bicarbonate when the stones were first reported to be uric acid (4), with no diminution in stone formation. The child has since been stone free for more than five years on allopurinol alone (10 mg/kg) without alkali (4). Another child was probably given antacid tablets prior to her presentation at the age of 19 months (5). One of the most recent cases (10) was treated with potassium citrate for a month presuming a uric acid stone, following the identification of a radiolucent stone by IVP and 'uric acid' crystals in the urine. IVP one month later demonstrated an increase in the filling defect (10). Allopurinol without alkali (10 or 5 mg/kg, dependent on renal function) has elimanted 2,8-DHA from the urine and with it any further stone formation in affected subjects to date (6).

The nephrotoxicity of 2,8-DHA has long been known from adenine loading studies in animals (3). The reason for the nephrotoxicity is the extreme insolubility of 2,8-DHA (approximately 1.5 mg/litre in water), fifty times less soluble than uric acid. Unlike uric acid,where a 12-fold increment occurs, the solubility of 2,8-DHA in urine is not significantly altered between pH 5.0 (2.7 mg/litre) and pH 7.4 (4.9 mg/litre) (13). Alkali will thus be ineffective (8) and the above results suggest its use may even be contra-indicated (6). However, urinary supersaturation with levels of 2,8-DHA up to 96 mg/litre has been reported during adenine loading studies (13). One untreated asymptomatic homozygote frequently excretes 2,8-DHA levels of this order (4). Varying ability to supersaturate the urine may thus explain the existence of asymptomatic homozygotes.

Yet another problem may be encountered in the treatment of patients in whom severe renal damage has developed prior to correct diagnosis, and applies too in both uric acid and 2,8-DHA stone formers. Here the allopurinol dose must be reduced because oxipurinol, the active metabolite *in vivo*, is reabsorbed by the kidney and retained in excess in renal failure. The effective circulating levels are thus higher and the dose must be reduced accordingly, and oxipurinol levels in plasma monitored if possible,with the dose adjusted to keep circulating levels below 100 μmol/litre (14). Oxipurinol will not only potentiate the action of immunosuppressive drugs such as azathioprine but can itself produce severe bone marrow depression (14).

Although most of the adenine excreted in the defect appears to be of endogenous origin, as indicated from the fairly constant excretion of adenine metabolites (20–30% of the total purine excretion) on a low purine intake (Table 2), a diet low in purine is advised. The severe clinical manifestation in one child (Table 1) from a commune consuming foods with a reputedly high adenine content, may have been aggravated by this diet (6). The source of the endogenous adenine production in APRT deficiency has been the subject of much speculation. Studies in intact and lysed cells from homozygotes (forming an effective adenine trap) have confirmed the insignificance of any pathway for the produc-

Table 2: The excretion of adenine metabolites compared to total oxypurine excretion (xanthine plus hypocanthine plus uric acid) in relatively constant proportion and increase with growth in four homozygotes [B. D. (3), F. Dh. (4), S. Rz. (5), Sk. B. (6)]. With the exception of F. Dh., who is untreated, all have been on allopurinol since the time of diagnosis (Table 1) and excrete adenine with only traces of 8-OH adenine and no 2,8-DHA.

urinary purine excretion (mmol/24 h) in APRT deficiency							
Patient		1975	1976	1977	1978	1979	1980
B.Dh.	Adenine compounds	.26	.30	.33	.56	.59	.60
	Total oxypurines	1.03	1.05	.88	1.68	2.4	2.24
	Adenine % total	25.2	28.6	37.5	33.3	24.6	26.8
F.Dh.	Adenine compounds		.43	.39	.51	.67	.64
	Total oxypurines		1.88	1.72	2.39	3.09	3.25
	Adenine % total		22.9	22.7	21.3	21.7	19.7
S.Rz.	Adenine compounds			.23	.27	.44	.30
	Total oxypurines			.82	.98	1.3	1.01
	Adenine % total			28.0	27.6	33.8	29.7
Sk.B.	Adenine compounds					.10	.14
	Total oxypurines					.37	.61
	Adenine % total					27.0	23.0

Total oxypurines: Adenine compounds + hypoxanthine + xanthine + uric acid

tion of adenine from adenosine in man (6). However, we have recently established significant adenine production in both these systems from 5'-methylthioadenisone by action of 5'-methylthioadenosine phosphorylase (Sahota et al in preparation for publication); the specific activity in lysates ranging from 6–10 nmol/mg Hb/h. This pathway has also been demonstrated recently in lymphocytes as well as other tissues (15). Adenine production as a by-product of the polyamine pathway (Fig. 1) thus seems the most likely *in vivo* source of the adenine excreted in APRT deficiency.

We do not yet know the real incidence of homozygosity for APRT deficiency. Four population studies suggest it may be high, since the incidence of heterozygosity is around 1 per hundred (6). Factors which could mask the real incidence are the wide spectrum of clinical expression (many will be unrecognised); the potentially lethal nature of the defect and/or the difficulties of diagnosis (many will be diagnosed and treated as uric acid stones); and the possibility of death *in utero* as suggested by the four spontaneous abortions in one family (4).

The prognosis in APRT deficiency clearly depends on the renal function at the time of diagnosis. This underlines the importance of early recognition and appropriate treatment. Allopurinol, – without alkali – will inhibit the formation of the nephrotoxic 2,8-DHA, and thus effectively prevent what should be an essentially benign disorder becoming a potentially lethal one. The long-term effect of allopurinol therapy with its potential for adenine accumulation, particularly in those cases with severe renal damage, remains to be established. All supposed uric acid stones should be submitted for analysis by special techniques to avoid any further confusion in the future.

References

1. Seegmiller, J.E.: Genetic defects in human purine metabolism leading to urolithiasis, in: Urolithiasis Research, H. Fleisch, W.G. Robertson, D.H. Smith, W. Vahlensieck (eds), New York, Plenum Press, 1976, p. 147–155.
2. Cartier, P., Hamet, M.: Une nouvelle maladie métabolique: le défecit complet en adénine-phosphoribosyltransférase avec lithiase de 2,8-dihydroxyadénine, C.R. Acad. Sci., Paris, **279:** 883, 1974.
3. Simmonds, H.A., Van Acker, K.J., Cameron, J.S., Snedden, W.: A new cause of urinary calculi: 2,8-dihydroxyadenine stones in supposed 'uric acid' crystalluria, in: Urolithiasis Research, H. Fleisch, W.G. Robertson, L.H. Smith, W. Vahlensieck (eds) New York, Plenum Press, 1976, p. 517–521.
4. Van Acker, K.J., Simmonds, H.A., Potter, C.F., Cameron, J.S.: Complete deficiency of adenine phosphoribosyltransferase. N. Engl. J. Med. **297:** 127, 1977.
5. Barratt, T.M., Simmonds, H.A. Cameron, J.S., Potter, C.F. Rose, G.A., Arkell, D.G., Williams, D.I.: Complete deficiency of adenine phosphoribosyltransferase, a third case presenting as renal stones in a young child. Arch. Dis. Child, **54:** 25, 1979.
6. Simmonds, H.A.: 2,8-dihydroxyadeninuria, or when is a uric acid stone not a uric acid stone? Clin. Nephrol **12:** 195, 1979.
7. Reveillaud, R.J., Daudon, M., Protat, M.F., Vincens, A., Graveleau, D.: Lithiase 2,8-dihydroxyadeninique: un nouveau cas dépisté par analyse infra-rouge. Nouv. Presse Med. **8:** 2965, 1979.
8. Cartier, P., Hamet, M., Vincens, A., Perignon, J.L.: Complete adenine phosphoribosyltransferase (APRT) deficiency in two siblings: report of a new case, in: Purine Metabolism in Man III, A. Rapado, R.W.E. Watts, C.H.M.M. de Bruyn (eds) Delete Izza New York, Plenum, 1980, p. 343.
9. Schabel, F., Doppler, W., Hirsch-Kauffmann, M., Glatzl, J., Schweiger, M., Berger, H., Heinz-Erian, P.: Hereditary deficiency of adenine phosphoribosyltransferase. Padiatr. u. Padol. **15:** 233, 1980.
10. Joost, J., Doppler, W.: The 2,8-dihydroxyadenine stone in childhood (in press).
11. Kuroda, M., Miki T., Kiyohara, H., Usami, M., Nakamura, T., Kotake, T., Takemoto, M., Sonoda, T.: Urolithiasis composed of 2,8-dihydroxyadenine due to partial deficiency of adenine phosphoribosyltransferase. Report of a case (author's transl.) Nippon Hinyokika Gakkal Azsshi 1980; **71(3):** 283–8.
12. Simmonds, H.A., Sahota, A., Potter, C.F., Cameron, J.S.: Purine metabolism and immunodeficiency: urinary purine excretion as a diagnostic screening test in adenosine deaminase and purine nucleoside phosphorylase deficiency. Clin. Sci. and Molec. Med. **54:** 579–584 (1978).
13. Peck, C.C., Bailey, F.J., Moore, G.L.: Enhanced solubility of 2,8-dihydroxyadenine (DOA) in human urine. Transfusion **17:** 383, 1977.
14. Cameron, J.S., and Simmonds, H.A.: Uric acid, gout and the kidney. J. Clin. Path. (In press).
15. Ferro, A.J., Vandenbark, A.A., Marchitto, K.: The role of 5'-methylthioadenosine phosphorylase in 5'-methylthioadenosinemediated inhibition of lymphocyte transformation. Biochim. Biophys. Acta., **588:** 294–301 (1979).

Author's address:

Dr. *H.A. Simmonds*
Guy's Hospital Medical School
Purine laboratory
London Bridge
London SE 1 9 RT
U. K.

Fortschritte der Urol. und Nephrol. 16, 58–65 (1981)
Steinkopff Verlag Darmstadt

Complete Adenine Phosphoribosyltransferase Deficiency with 2,8-Dihydroxyadenine Stone Formation

J. Joost[1], F. Schabel[2], and W. Doppler[3]

1 Department of Urology
2 Department of Pediatrics
3 Institut für Biochemie (Nat. Fak.)
Universität Innsbruck, Austria

In 1968 Kelley (1) described for the first time a patient with a partial adenine phosphoribosyltransferase (APRT) deficiency. Since that time many families have been found with this abnormality in the heterozygous state. Though in some families gout could be detected, no consistent correlation with gout or hyperuricemia was noted. No clinical disorder has yet been found to be consistently associated with a partial deficiency of APRT. The incidence in the population has been estimated to be 0.5 to 1% (2).
In 1974 Cartier (3) was the first to describe a complete deficiency of APRT. Since that time 9 children have been described, 4 in London, 3 in Paris, and 2 in Innsbruck (4, 5, 6). As a consequence of the complete deficiency of APRT the following abnormalities in purine metabolism can be found (Fig. 1). In the absence of APRT, adenine cannot be reutilized. 2,8-dihydroxyadenine (DOA) ist formed, because adenine now becomes available for oxidation by xanthine oxidase. High levels of adenine and DOA are found in the urine. The clinical consequence of homozygocity for this enzyme defect is presented in two case reports.

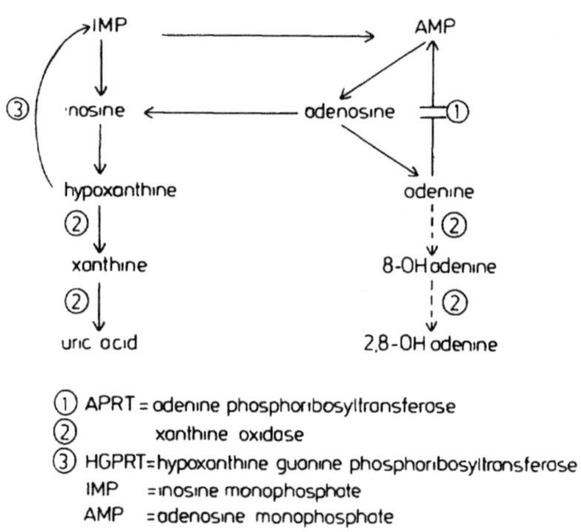

Fig. 1: Purine metabolism.

Case report 1

H.F. was born in 1967. At the age of 17 months the patient was admitted to the pediatric department with acute renal failure. The initial treatment consisted of peritoneal dialysis.

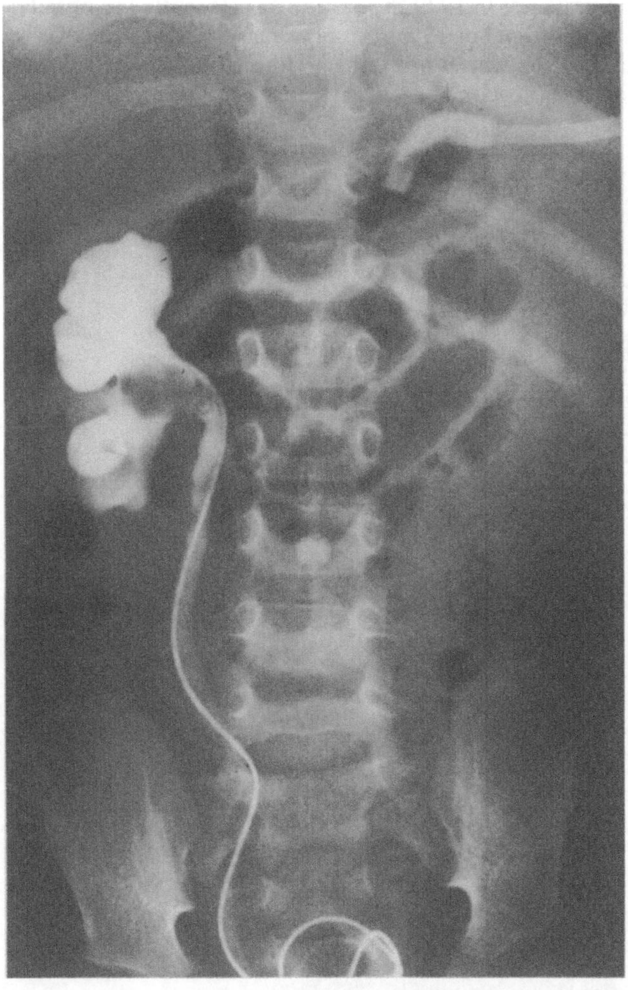

Fig. 2: Retrograde pyelography showing stones and excessice hydronephrosis.

In the IVP no exact diagnosis was made. A retrograde pyelography was performed and showed radiolucent stones on both sides with excessive hydronephrosis (Fig. 2). The child then underwent many operations for stone removal and loop nephrostomies were performed on both sides. The chemical analysis of the stones revealed urates. The child was kept in hospital and was discharged in 1969 (Fig. 3). Afterwards irregular checkups took place. In 1977 he was readmitted to hospital. At that time creatinine was raised to 2.2 mg% and creatinine clearance was 30 ml/min/1.73 m^2. The urine was sterile and the IVP showed small kidneys on both sides with loss of parenchyma (Fig. 4). No stones could be detected. The next inpatient control in 1978 showed no significant change. In the same year complete APRT deficiency was detected by measuring the activity of erythrocyte hemolysates. One year later in 1979 the patient was readmitted to hospital with renal insufficiency, a creatinine level of 15 mg%, and a creatinine clearance of 3.9 ml/min/1.73 m^2 was found. Hemodialysis had to be performed and the patient was included in a dialysis program. He is now on the waiting list for renal transplantation.

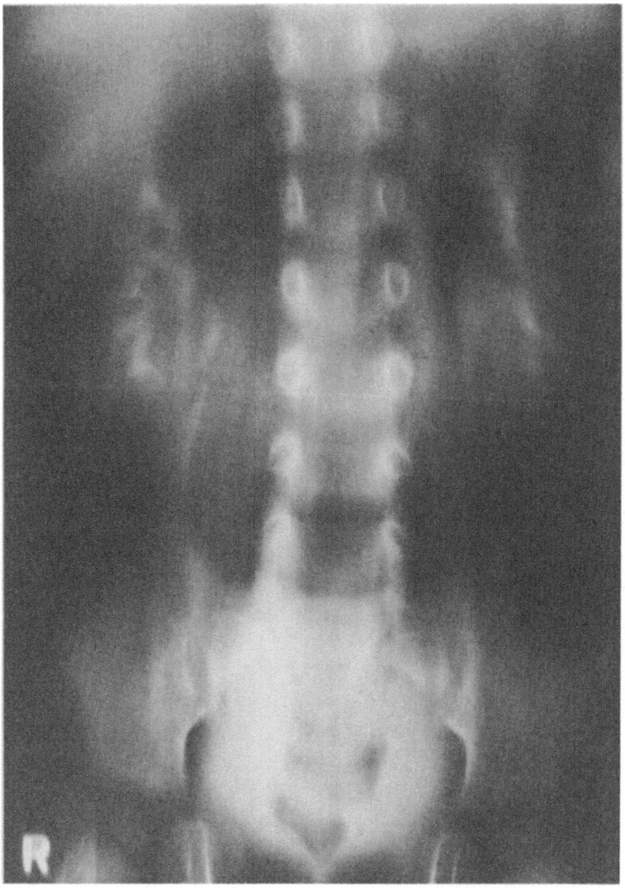

Fig. 3: IVP after operations for stone removal and loop nephrostomies.

Case report 2

Th.M. was born in 1971. He was admitted to hospital because of recurrent right flank pain and hematuria. In the IVP a filling defect in the right pelvis could be seen. Uric acid was normal in serum and urine. Therapy consisted of alkalization by potassium citrate presuming a uric acid stone. The control IVP one month later clearly demonstrated an increase of the filling defect. Ultrasound confirmed the diagnosis of a stone in the right

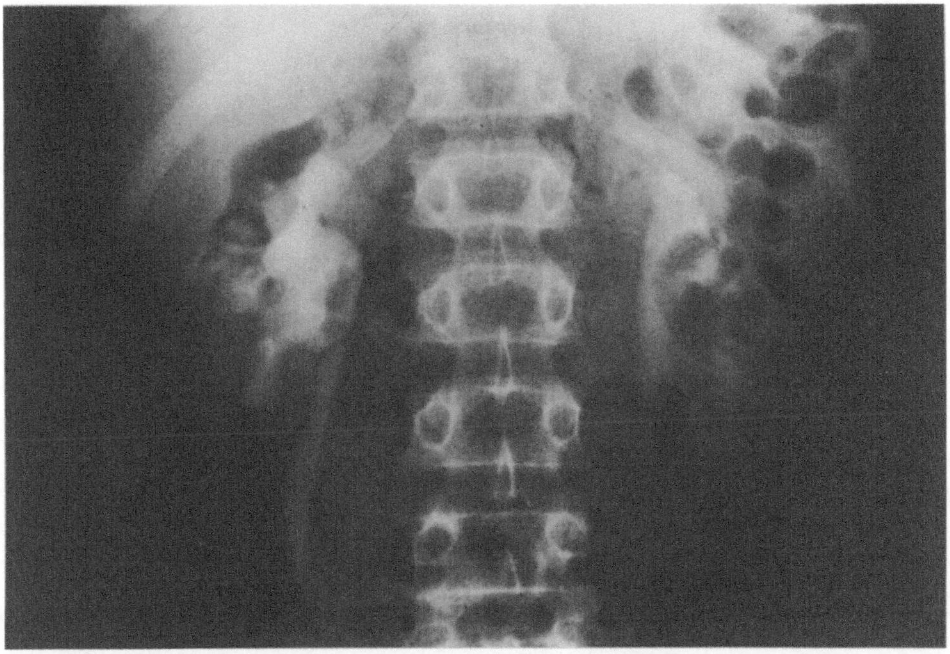

Fig. 4: IVP showing small kidneys with loss of parenchyma.

pelvis. The calculus was removed by pyelotomy. Parts of the stones were analyzed chemically and by X-ray diffraction. Chemical analysis revealed a uric acid stone whereas X-ray diffraction showed DOA as the only compound. An exact microscopic analysis of the urine showed typical round brown crystals. To prove the APRT deficiency an enzyme test was performed. After diagnosis had been confirmed, therapy consisted of 50 mg allopurinol twice daily. One year later the boy had a normal IVP and normal isotope clearance of the kidneys.

The clinical consequence of homozygosity for this enzyme defect is given by the increased formation of DOA. The high excretion of this insoluble substance leads to crystalluria and stone formation. Only two of the nine children had crystalluria, whereas all others formed urinary stones. Solubility studies of DOA in human urine have been carried out by Peck (7). He determined the basal solubility (solubility product), which is approximately 4.97 mg/liter at a pH of 7.8. The metastable range seems to be at least up to 10 times higher than the solubility product. Within the physiological pH-range no significant solubility increase occurs. This is quite in contrast to uric acid, which displays pH-dependence solubility. In 3 children the amount of DOA in the urine is reported and was between 20 and 60 mg per 24 hours, measured by HPLC. One asymptomatic child with crystalluria had about the same values as the other two, who formed stones. Up to now no work has been done on inhibitors or solubilizing substances in the urine for DOA. The crystals are round, brown, and in our studied case measured up to 5 μm. They form bigger aggregations and sometimes seem to be connected by bridges (Figs. 5,6,7). The

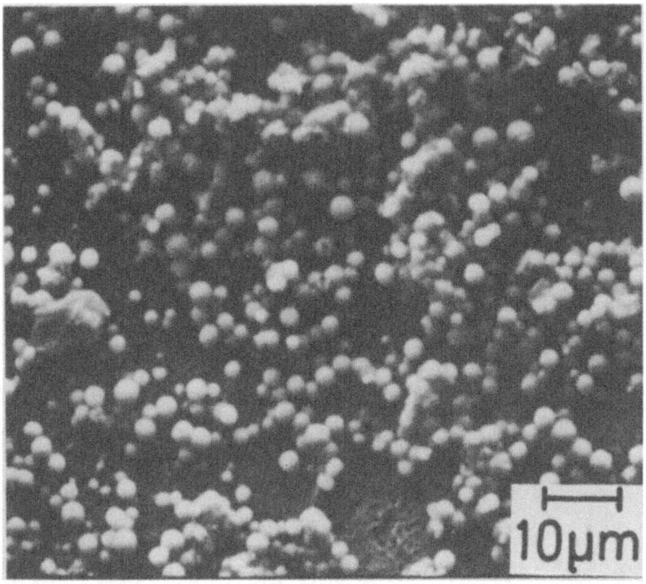

Fig. 5: 2,8-dihydroxyadenine crystals.

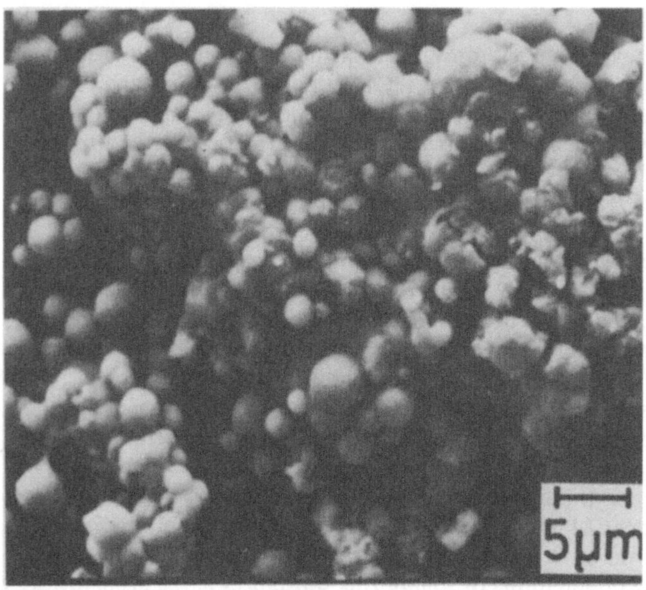

Fig. 6: 2,8-dihydroxyadenine crystals.

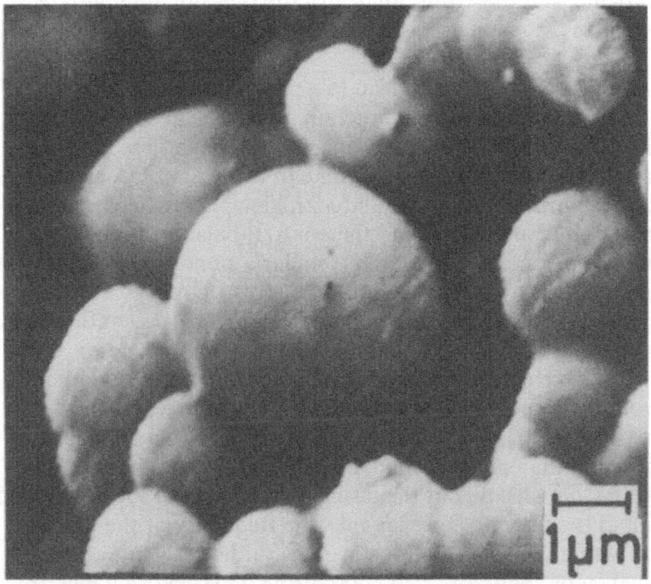

Fig. 7: 2,8-dyhydroxyadenine crystals.

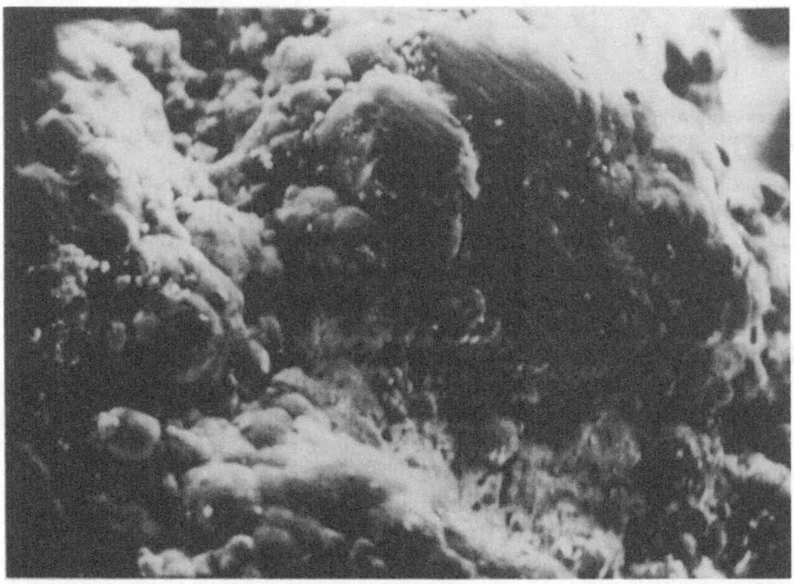

Fig. 8: SEM picture of 2,8-dihydroxyadenine stone surface.

stones are grayish-blue and friable, and therefore can be macroscopically differentiated from uric acid. SEM pictures of the stone surface show again the round crystals by which the stone is formed (Fig. 8).

The high excretion of the insoluble DOA may also lead to a progressive renal disease. Four of the reported children have reduced kidney function, in two in an advanced stage. Renal failure seems not only to be a result of obstruction and subsequent infection. As long ago as 1898, Minkowski (8) showed by feeding adenine to dogs that DOA crystals are deposited in the renal parenchyma and lead to an interstitial nephritis. Simmonds (4) performed a renal biopsy in one child and also found these intratubular crystals. Up to now it is not clear if asymptomatic homozygotes with crystalluria alone might also develop into a chronic renal insufficiency by the nephrotoxicity of DOA.

The inheritance of this enzyme defect is an autosomal recessive trait. This is confirmed by the pedigree of our first patient (H.F.) (Fig. 9). The father and mother are heterozygotes with a reduced APRT activity. Two children are normal and two others are also heterozygotes. The APRT activity in the propositus is less than 1%. Not quite clear is the pedigree of our second case (Th.M.) (Fig. 9). He also has an activity of less than 1%. Three of the children are heterozygotes and the youngest child, born in Oct. 1980 is normal. The mother has an incomplete APRT deficiency, but the husband has a normal activity. Blood matches seem to exclude him as the father of our patient. The frequency of the heterozygotes has been determined with an incidence of one in 233. For homozygotes there should be an estimated frequency of about 1 per 200 000 births. This relatively high frequency compared to only 9 diagnosed cases is indicative that this disease may not be recognized properly in urological practice today.

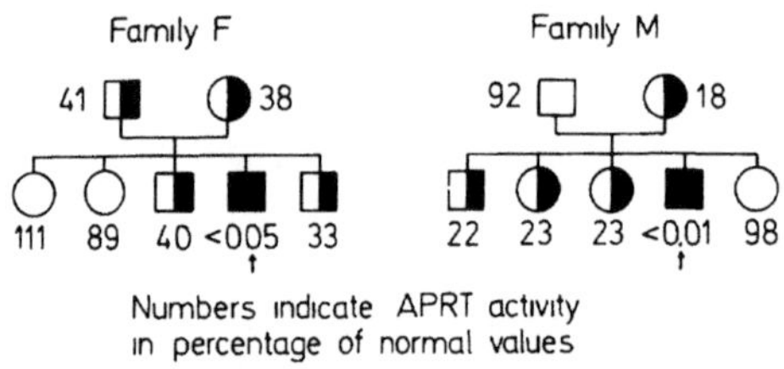

Fig. 9: Predigree of Case Report 1. and 2.

In any child presenting with obstructive symptoms by radiolucent stones the possibility of APRT deficiency should be considered, especially if the patient has a normal content of urate in serum and urine. When uric acid stones are identified by routine, chemical analysis, then additional confirmatory tests should be performed since there is no possibility of distinguishing between uric acid and DOA in a simple chemical analysis. Only a crystallographic method as for instance X-ray diffraction or infrared spectrophotometry detects the DOA compound (Fig. 10). As already mentioned, these stones are grayish blue and more friable than uric acid. Confirmation of the diagnosis provides the measurement of the APRT activity in erythrocyte hemolysates (3). All other members of a family should be screened for the APRT deficiency, because some might only have asymptomatic crystalluria.

A very simple approach to the treatment of this disease is made possible by the fact that xanthine oxidase is responsible for generating DOA. The xanthine oxidase inhibitor allopurinol reduces the formation of DOA. Stones which do not pass spontaneously have to be removed by operation or instrumentation. As already described dissolution of the stone is not possible. The solubility in urine is significantly increased at a pH of 8.5 and

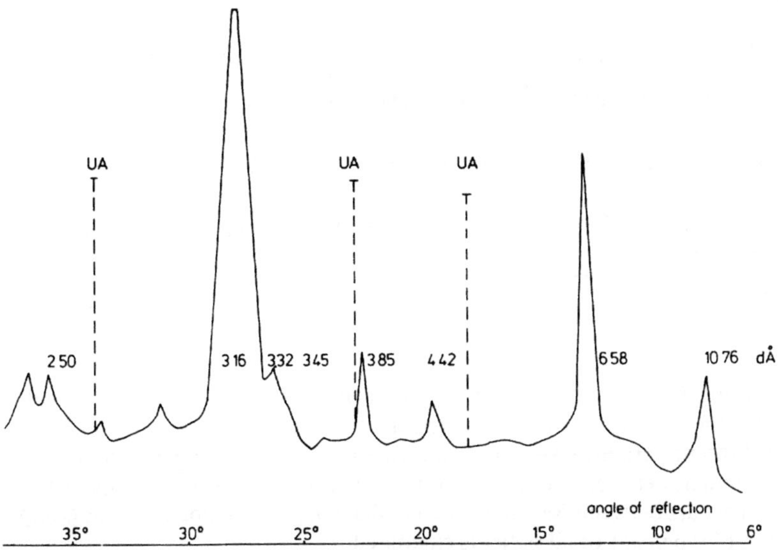

Fig. 10: X-ray diffractogram of 2,8-dihydroxyadenine. UA, uric acid.

higher. These are intolerable values for humans. A diet low in purines reduces the total amount of adenine and its metabolites in urine (9). Nothing is known to date about the treatment of asymptomatic homozygotes.

References

1. Kelley, W.N., Levy, R.I., Rosenbloom, F.M., Henderson, J.F. and Seegmiller, J.E.: Adenine phosphoribosyltransferase deficiency: A previously undescribed genetic defect in man. J. Clin. Invest. **47**: 2281, 1968.
2. Johnson, L.A., Gordon, R.B. and Emmerson, B.T.: Adenine phosphoribosyltransferase: A simple spectaphotometry assay and the incidence of mutation in the normal population. Biochemical Genetics, **15**: 265, 1977.
3. Cartier, R. and Hamet, M.: Une nouvelle maladie metabolique: Le deficit complet en adenine phosphoribosyltransferase avec lithiase de 2,8-dihydroxyadenine. C.R. Acad. Sci. **297**: 883, 1974.
4. Simmonds, H.A.: 2,8-Dihydroxyadeninuria–or when is a uric acid stone not a uric acid stone? Clin. Nephrol, **12**: 195, 1979.
5. Schabel, F., Doppler, W., Hirsch-Kauffmann, M., Schweiger, M., Berger, H. and Heinz-Frian, P.: Hereditary deficiency of adenine phosphoribosyltransferase. Pàdiat. Pàdol., **15**: 233, 1980.
6. Joost, J. and Doppler, W.: The 2,8-dihydroxyadenine stone in childhood. (in press)
7. Peck, C.C., Bailey, F.J. and Moore, G.L.: Enhanced solubility of 2,8-dihydroxyadenine (DOA) in human urine. Transfusion, **17**: 383, 1977.
8. Minkowski, O.: Untersuchungen zur Physiologie und Pathologie der Harnsäure bei Säugetieren. Archiv f. experiment. Pathol. u. Pharmakol., **41**: 375, 1898.
9. Barratt, T.M., Simmonds, H.A., Cameron, J.S., Potter, C.F., Rose, G.A., Arkell, D.g. and Williams, D.I.: Complete deficiency of adenine phosphoribosyltransferase. Arch. Dis. Childh., **54**: 25, 1979.

Author's address:

Dr. *J. Joost*
Urologische Universitatsklinik Innsbruck
6010 Innsbruck
Austria

Fortschritte der Urol. und Nephrol. **16**, 66–69 (1981)
Steinkopff Verlag Darmstadt

Idiopathic Uric Acid Lithiasis – Some Less Known Epidemiologie and Metabolic Findings

D. Scholz[1], P. O. Schwille[1], W. Engelhardt[1], and A. Sigel[2]

Mineral Metabolism and Hormone Research Laboratory,
Departments of Surgery[1] and Urology[2]
Universität Erlangen, West Germany

In patients with urolithiasis, stones composed of uric acid are the second most frequent stone species following calcium-containing stones. In our outpatient clinic about 17 percent of all urolithiasis patients have uric acid stones (1). Whereas calcium-containing stones are most frequent between the ages of 36 to 55 years, the maximum frequency of uric acid stones occurs between 56 and 65 years. Males are predominant in this group and comprise about 70 percent of all patients examined.
To establish metabolic criteria relevant for the process of diagnostic decision making, we studied patients with mineralogically proven uric acid lithiasis, but without clinically manifest symptoms of gout (= idiopathic uric acid lithiasis).

Material and Methods

24 men and 6 women with idiopathic uric acid lithiasis were included in the study. Their ages varied between 40 and 63 years. As a control group, age-matched healthy members of the hospital and their relatives were investigated. Our guidelines on how to work on stone patients under ambulatory conditions, i. e., without dietary prescriptions, have been described earlier (2, 3). All analyses followed conventional methods. Results are indicated as x ± 1 standard error (table 2) and x ± 1 standard deviation (fig. 1) in the case of normal distributions, otherwise as median and the range of individual values.

Table 2: Age, sex distribution, and body weight of healthy controls and patients with idiopathic uric acid stones and the stone history of the latter. Values represent median with the respective range, except column with sex distribution. N = number of cases. A.: $p < 0.01$ versus healthy controls.

	Age years	Sex ♂ N	Sex ♀ N	Body weight kg	Stone frequency	Operative removals	Spontaneous passages
Healthy controls; N = 20	51 40 - 63	12	8	70 57 - 100	- -	- -	- -
Idiopathic uric acid stone formers; N = 30	53 39 - 69	24	6	79[A] 56 - 115	3 1 - 23	[illegible] 0 - 2	3 0 - 22

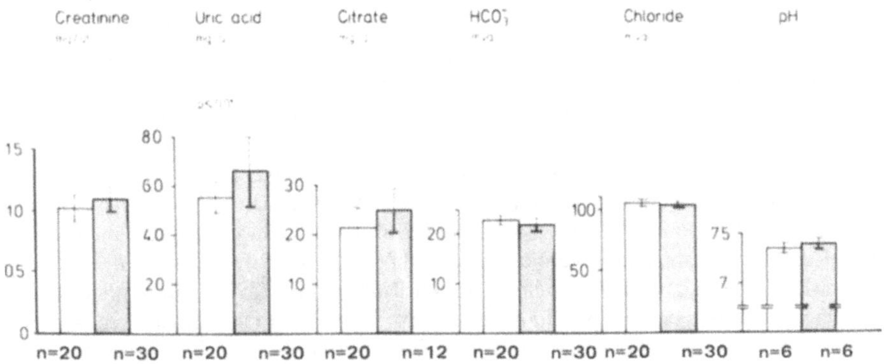

Fig. 1: Mean serum values of healthy controls (⊓) and idiopathic uric acid stone formers (▥). T = 1 standard deviation of mean; HCO_3 = bicarbonate; n = number of observations.

Results

Clinical data (table 1): patients with idiopathic uric acid lithiasis usually have a higher body weight ($p < 0.05$). On average each patient formed 3 stones in the history, which almost all passed spontaneously, i. e., only 3 percent of the stones formed were removed by operation. In contrast, in patients with calcium oxalate renal stones, who also formed 3 stones on average in the history, in 30 percent of all stones surgical removal was necessary. This peculiar finding may focus attention on the rather smooth surface of uric acid stones, thereby facilitating spontaneous passage through the urinary tract.

Blood values (fig. 1): creatinine is normal, uric acid slightly elevated $p < 0.01$ in the median values are 5.83 (controls) and 6.78 (patients) mg/dl. The median citrate is 2.15 (controls) and 2.45 (patients) mg/dl (not significant). According to our data on chloride, bicarbonate, and capillary blood pH, the blood acid–base status of the patients is not disturbed.

Table 1: Indirect and direct parameters of parathyroid gland function in serum and 2-hr-fasting urine (NcAMP).
Values represent x ± 1 standard error (normal distribution), otherwise median and range; ( ) = number of observations. $Protein_T$ = total protein, $Calcium_T$ = total calcium, $Calcium_I$ = ionized calcium, $Magnesium_T$ = total magnesium, $Magnesium_F$ = free ultrafiltrable magnesium, TmP = phosphate threshold concentration, PTH = parathyroid hormone, NcAMP = nephrogenous cyclic adenosine monophosphate. A: $p < 0.05$; B: $p < 0.01$; C: $p < 0.001$ versus controls.

	$Protein_T$ g/dl	$Calcium_T$ mg/dl	$Calcium_I$ mg/dl	$Magnesium_T$ mg/dl	$Magnesium_F$ mg/dl	Phosphate mg/dl	TmP mg/dl	PTH pg-Eq/ml	NcAMP
Healthy controls; n = 20	7.3 ± 0.1	9.84 ± 0.07	4.45 ± 0.11	2.15 ± 0.04	1.48 ± 0.02	3.62 ± 0.1	3.75 2.75-5.00	174 <150-630 (12)	2.24 -0.58-6.28 (17)
Idiopathic uric acid stone formers, n = 30	7.5 ± 0.1^A	9.87 ± 0.07	4.66 ± 0.10	1.96 ± 0.04^C	1.37 ± 0.03^B	2.96 ± 0.1^C	3.30^C 1.60-4.55	<150 <150-547 (8)	1.53 -0.03-2.83 (12)

Values in the urine (fig. 2): the values, except pH, were corrected for 1.73 m^2 body surface. The daily excretion of calcium on average is slightly lower in patients than in controls ($p < 0.05$). The median values are 142 (patients) and 190 (controls) mg. The uric acid excretion of the patients does not differ from age-matched controls: the median value of controls is 526, of patients 505 mg. Only one case with a uric acid excretion above our control range (= interdecile range 80) was found. The citrate excretion, which was based on the enzymatic citrate measurement (4), is clearly low in patients: the median value of controls is 585, of patients 308 mg ($p < 0.01$). Urinary tract and renal tissue infection as a cause of the low citrate values were excluded according to routine clinical investigations and the rather low urinary pH (see below). In addition, patients with idiopathic uric acid lithiasis have a distinctly lower pH than controls ($p < 0.05$), which has been recognized for a long time. The mean value of controls is 5.78, of patients 5.55. Similar values are found in the 2-hr-fasting urine, i. e., unchanged uric acid excretion and a more acidic pH, but a normal citrate excretion (P.O. Schwille, D. Scholz; unpublished data).

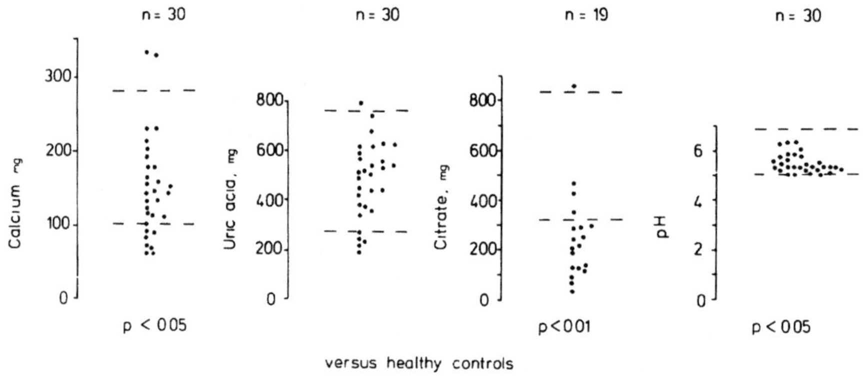

Fig. 2: Values in the daily urine of patients with idiopathic uric acid lithiasis. Hatched lines represent 2 standard deviations (pH) or interdecile range 80 (calcium, uric acid, citrate) of healthy controls (n = 20); n = number of observations.

Parameters of parathyroid gland function (table 2): total serum protein is elevated in the patients ($p < 0.05$), but total and ionized calcium are unchanged. Magnesium (total, free filtrable fraction), phosphate and phosphate treshold concentration are low ($p < 0.001$ and $p < 0.01$ resp.). Serum parathyroid hormone was determined by an amino- and carboxyl-terminal assay, using antibody 211/41 Wellcome (final dilution 1:150 000) and highly purified bovine gland extract for standard and tracer preparations. According to our previous investigations this assay system detects intact human parathyroid hormone and circulating parathyroid hormone fragments (5). Rather low parathyroid hormone values are found in the patients, although a coincidence between uric acid lithiasis and primary hyperparathyroidism was reported earlier (6). Urinary cyclic adenosine monophosphate (2-hr-fasting urine), presented as the nephrogenous part, is slightly lower in patients than in controls, and this observation agrees well with the low serum parathyroid hormone, but not with the low serum phosphate.

Conclusions

Patients with idiopathic uric acid lithiasis are predominantly men, have a higher age than patients with calcium-containing renal stones, and are often overweight. In the majority of cases uric acid stones pass spontaneously and rarely need surgical removal. In these patients an only moderate hyperuricemia is found, while the urinary uric acid excretion does not differ from age-matched controls. The cause for the too high titrable acidity in the urine of these patients is uncertain, especially as urinary ammonium excretion is controversially judged (7, 8) and as more specific investigations on acid base metabolism are lacking. A possible etiological relationship between the development of uric acid lithiasis and the low urinary citrate excretion may be considered, especially as citrate is much higher in controls with urinary pH in the same order of magnitude. Also the manner in which a low parathyroid gland function might contribute to uric acid stone-forming processes is not understood on the basis of current knowledge of mineral metabolism (= low urinary calcium and relatively high phosphate) in this subgroup of idiopathic (= metabolically induced) urolithiasis.

Acknowledgments

The paper was supported in part by a grant from Universitätsbund Erlangen.

References

1. Scholz, D., Schwille, P.O., Ulbrich, D., Bausch, W.M., Sigel, A.: Composition of renal stones and their frequency in a stone clinic: relationship to parameters of mineral metabolism in serum and urine. Urol. Res. 7: 161–170 (1979).
2. Scholz, D., Schwille, P.O., Sigel, A.: Zur metabolischen Klassifikation und Metaphylaxe der häufigsten Lithiasisformen. Urologe A 19: 202–206 (1980).
3. Schwille, P.O., Scholz, D., Sigel, A.: Urolithiasis–ein Überblick zur Pathophysiologie, Diagnostik und Therapie. W. klin. Wochenschr. 92: 411–420 (1980).
4. Schwille, P.O., Scholz, D., Paulus, M., Engelhardt, W., Sigel, A.: Citrate in daily and fasting urine. Results of controls, patients with recurrent idiopathic calcium urolithiasis, and primary hyperparathyroidism. Invest. Urol. 16: 457–462 (1979).
5. Schwille, P.O., Scholz, D.: Cyclic nucleotides and related variables in urolithiasis. In: Smith, L.H., Robertson, W.G., Finlayson, B. (eds): Urolithiasis. Clinical and Basic Research, Plenum Press, New York, 835–839 (1981).
6. Scott, J.T., Dixon, A.St., Bywaters, E.G.: Association of hyperuricemia and gout with hyperparathyroidism. Br. Med. J. 5390: 1070–1077 (1964).
7. Gutman, A.B., Yü, T.F.: Renal regulation of uric acid secretion in normal and gouty man: modifications by uricosuric agents, Bull. N.Y. Acad. Med. 34: 287–293 (1958).
8. Wrong, O.: Urinary hydrogen ion excretion in patients with uric acid calculi. Proceed. Royal Soc. Med. 59: 27–34 (1966).

Author's address:

Dieter Scholz, MD
University Hospital
Maximiliansplatz
8520 Erlangen
Germany

Fortschritte der Urol. und Nephrol. 16, 70–74 (1981)
Steinkopff Verlag Darmstadt

The Contribution of Dietary Purines to Urinary Urate Excretion in Gouty and Renal Stone Patients

A. Halabe, R. Samuel, U. A. Liberman, and O. Sperling

Metabolic Unit and Department of Clinical Biochemistry,
Beilinson Medical Center, Tel-Aviv
University School of Medicine, Petah-Tikva, Israel

Hyperuricosuria is a major etiological factor in uric acid lithiasis. In addition, there is evidence for an etiological role of hyperuricosuria in calcium oxalate stone formation (1, 2). Indeed, in our stone clinic, a high proportion of hyperuricosuria was also noticed among the patients with calcium urolithiasis. Since the hyperuricosuria in our stone clinic patients was established on the basis of urate determination on urine collections obtained on a regular home diet, the possibility of dietary hyperuricosuria was raised. We have therefore evaluated the contribution of dietary purine intake to uric acid excretion in our stone patients under controlled dietary conditions.

69 hyperuricosuric male patients, 30 to 65 years of age, suffering from gout and urolithiasis, were studied for two weeks in a metabolic ward. During the first week, their diet contained 90 mg purines, 95 g proteins, 48 g fat, and 280 g carbohydrates, a total of 1900 calories per day. During the second week an isocaloric diet containing 20 mg purines, 80 g protein, 52 g fat, and 280 g carbohydrates per day was given. Urines were collected daily for the last 4 days of each week. Creatinine and uric acid were determined in blood and urine by colorimetric methods (3).

Results and Discussion

On the basis of the results obtained during the first period, the patients were divided into 3 groups: normouricemic–normouricosuric, hyperuricemic–normouricosuric, and hyperuricemic–hyperuricosuric (Table 1).

Lowering purine intake in the second week from 90 to 20 mg/day resulted in a significant decrease in each group in both serum urate level and urinary urate excretion (Figs. 1 and

Table 1: Patient groups studied

	Patients	No.	Serum urate* (mg/dl)	Urinary urate excretion* (mg/24 h)
I	Normouricemic–normouricosuric	30	6.7 ± 0.94	606 ± 80
II	Hyperuricemic–normouricosuric	19	8.9 ± 0.76	604 ± 99
III	Hyperuricemic–hyperuricosuric	20	8.4 ± 1.16	893 ± 90

* Values represent averages of uric acid values obtained on each of the last 4 days during a week on a diet containing 90 mg purines/day.

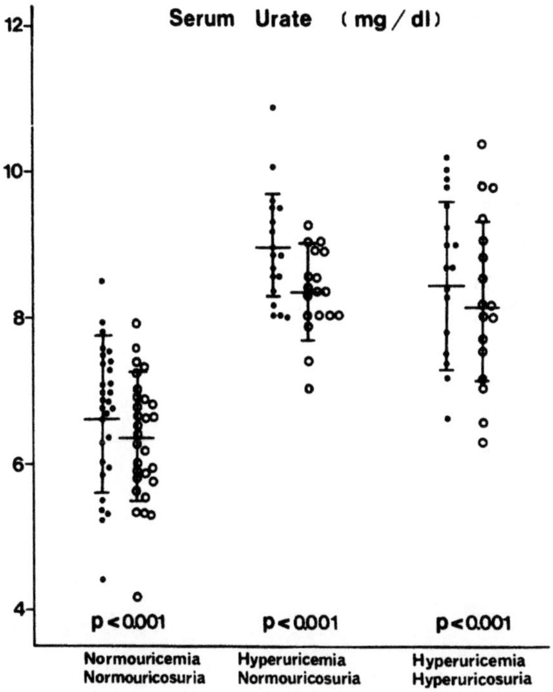

Fig. 1: Effect of low purine intake (20 mg/day) on serum urate level.

2). The decrease in urinary urate excretion was significant when expressed as mg/24 h (Fig. 2a), as mg/mg creatinine (Fig. 2b), and as mg/100 ml GFR (Fig. 2c). The decrease in urinary urate excretion was greater than that in serum urate level, resulting in a decrease in renal urate clearance values in all groups studied (Fig. 3).

The results of this study show that primary purine overproduction is rare among hyperuricosuric stone patients. This is based on the finding that transfer from a home diet to a diet containing 90 mg purines per day resulted in the disappearance of the hyperuricosuria in 49 out of the 69 patients studied and that lowering purine intake to 20 mg/day resulted in a further reduction in urate excretion, reaching normal levels in most of the patients. On this low purine intake only 6 out of the original 69 hyperuricosuric patients had urate excretion values compatible with overproduction. It is of interest that 4 of these 6 apparently overproducing patients were found to be affected with compensated hemolytic syndromes, representing secondary metabolic hyperuricosuria. (Liberman et al, in this workshop).

The results of this study indicate that excessive purine intake is a major cause for hyperuricosuria among stone patients. Therefore, restriction of dietary purines is of therapeutic value in the treatment of nephrolithiasis.

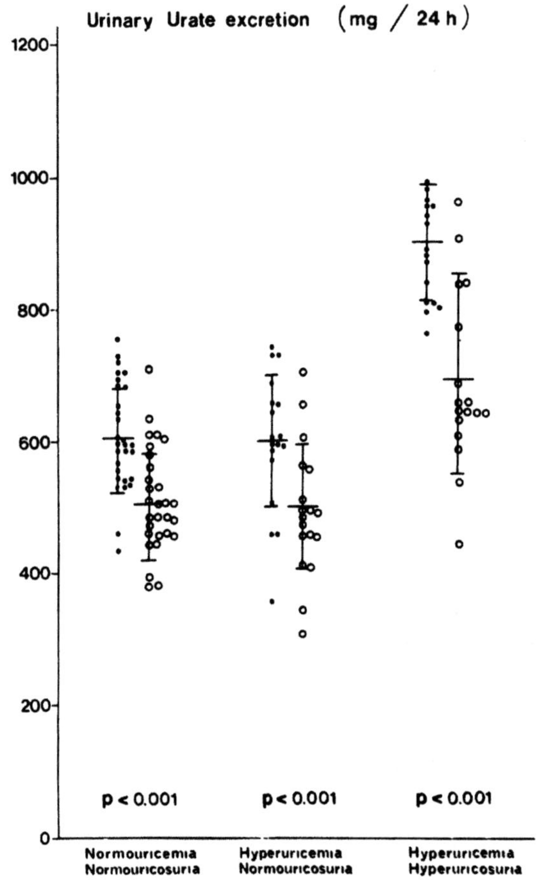
Urinary Urate excretion (mg / 24 h)
1200
1000
800
600
400
200
0
p < 0.001
p < 0.001
p < 0.001
Normouricemia Normouricosuria
Hyperuricemia Normouricosuria
Hyperuricemia Hyperuricosuria

2a

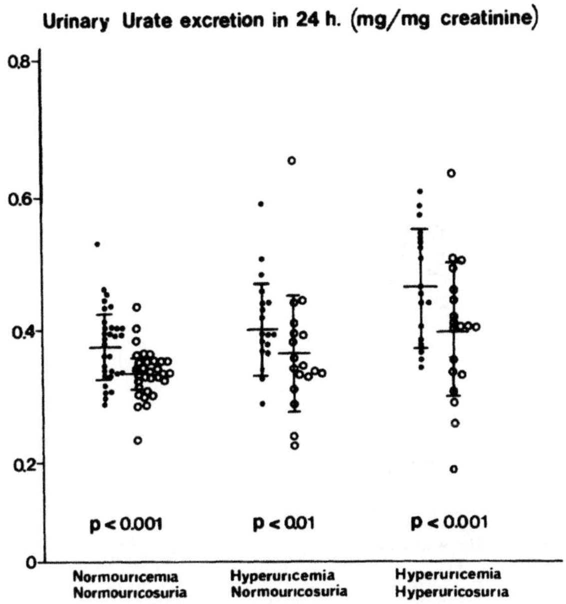

2b

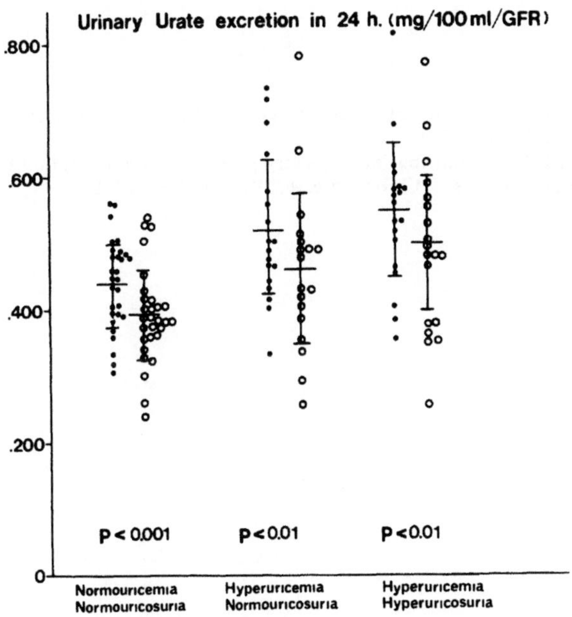

2c

Fig. 2: Effect of low purine intake (20 mg/day) on urinary urate excretion: expressed as mg/24 h (a); as mg/mg creatinine (b); and as mg/100 ml GFR (c).

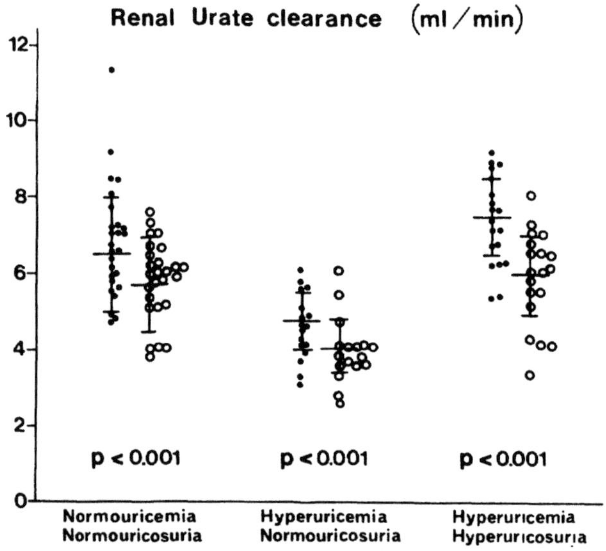

Fig. 3: Effect of low purine intake (20 mg/day) on renal urate clearance.

References

1. Coe, F.C. and Kavalach, A.G.: Hypercalciuria and hyperuricosuria in patients with calcium nephrolithiasis. New Eng. J. Med., **291**: 1344–1350 (1974).
2. Coe, F.C., Moran, E. and Kavalach, A.G.: The contribution of dietary purine over–consumption to hyperuricosuria in calcium oxalate stone formers. J. Chron. Disease, **29**: 793–800 (1976).
3. Technicon AutoAnalyzer methodology.

Author's address

Dr. *A. Halabe*
Beilinson Medical Center
Metabolic Unit
Petah-Tikva
Israel

Fortschritte der Urol. und Nephrol. **16**, 75–80 (1981)
Steinkopff Verlag Darmstadt

Results of Examination in Renal Stone formers after Purine Load

B. Lux, J. Braun, and P. May

Urologische Klinik und Institut für Laboratoriumsmedizin des Allgemeinen Krankenhauses Bamberg, Akademisches Lehrkrankenhaus der Universität Erlangen, West Germany

It is known, that uric acid seems to be important in the formation of calcium oxalate stones. Robertson has shown in his model of stone formation the decrease of urinary inhibitory activity with high concentrations of uric acid. Thus the effective concentrations of the acid mucopolysaccharide fraction of urine may be reduced, which should favor the risk of stone formation. According to the literature (Table 1), hyperuricosuria is found in 15–40% of all patients with calcium oxalate stones.

Table 1: Frequency of hyperuricosuria in clacium oxalate stones (literature)

author	year	hyperuricosuria
Grob	1975	27%
Hodgkinson	1976	20%
Hartung	1977	♂ 40%
		♀ 32%
Braun	1977	32%
Matouschek	1979	17%
May	1980	28%

Ohlenschläger and Ulbrich suggested an oral purine load test as diagnostic for latent disorders in metabolism of uric acid and gout. Like Bach and Schneeberger we have tried to clarify whether a latent disorder of the metabolism of uric acid can also be found in oxalate stone formers, in order to recognize a possible risk factor for stone formation, and also whether a hyperuricemia or a hyperuricosuria is present in the routine examination of lithogenetic working substances.

Performance

The examinations were carried out with 9 healthy volunteers, 17 patients with pure calcium oxalate stones, and 11 patients with mixed calcium oxalate calculi. In all patients the serum uric acid was normal; however, in some patients with mixed calcium oxalate stones the uric acid excretion was higher.
After evaluation of the normal values in serum and 24-hour urine the patients recived 2 g purine base capsules with breakfast, containing the same amount of adenine and

guanine (*Harnsäurebelastungstest,* Fa. Dr. K. Fresenius, Oberursel/Taunus, West Germany). Subsequently for a period of 2 days blood was taken every 12 hours and 24 hour urine samples were collected twice. The purine load test was only performed in patients with a normal kidney function, proved with creatinine ≦ 1.2 mg/dl or creatinine clearance of more than 80 ml/min. The evaluation of the mean value significances was carried out by the U test according to Wilcoxon, Man, and Whithey. Instead of the usual standard deviation we used the MDM = mean deviation from the mean, which in accordance with Sachs is better than the standard deviation for considering small groups or if extreme values are suspected.

Results

In Table 2 can be seen the mean values of serum uric acid 12, 24, 36, and 48 hours after purine load. The uric acid increases in the normal group, but this increase is not significant against the basic value. On the contrary there is a significant increase in both patient groups during the first 24 hours after purine load, which in the mixed stone group had already reached the maximum after 12 hours, because of the significance limits. In the patients with pure calcium oxalate stones the maximum value was only reached after 24 hours, which is significantly different to the base value at the 0.5% level. Between both patient groups there is only a significance of p ≦ 0.05 after 24 and 36 hours.

Table 2: Purine load: serum uric acid (mg/dl)

	basal	12 h	24 h	36 h	48 h
controls (n = 9) x̄ ± MDM signific.	 5.3 ± 0.78	 6.13 ± 0.53 n. s.	 6.18 ± 0.67 n. s.	 5.40 ± 0.48 n. s.	 5.60 ± 0.53 n. s.
mixed ca. ox. (n = 11) x̄ ± MDM signific.	 4.26 ± 0.72	 5.29 ± 0.74 s. ≦ 1%	 5.17 ± 0.56 s. ≦ 2.5%	 4.56 ± 0.56 n. s.	 4.68 ± 0.55 n. s.
pure ca. ox. (n = 17) x̄ ± MDM signific.	 4.84 ± 0.85	 5.85 ± 0.94 s. ≦ 2.5%	 6.05 ± 0.95 s. ≦ 0.5%	 5.43 ± 1.04 n. s.	 5.43 ± 0.88 n. s.
signific. mixed-pure ca. oxalate	n. s.	n. s.	s. ≦ 5.0%	s. ≦ 5.0%	n. s.

MDM = mean deviation from the mean

The urinary uric acid concentration is inversely proportional to the serum values (Table 3). On the first day after purine load there is a high significant increase with p ≦ 0.005 in the control group; on the second day a high excretion of only small significance can be seen. On the other hand on both days the increase of the uric acid concentration in the mixed stone group is not significantly different from the base value; however it remains at the same level as on the first day. In the patients with pure calcium oxalate stones a high significant increase of uric acid excretion on the first day is also found, followed by a decrease, which is still significant compared with the base value at the 0.5% level, so that in both groups of stone formers a reduction of delayed elimination of uric acid can be assumed.

Table 3: Urinary uric acid concentration and uric acid clearance rate after purine load

	urinary uric acid (mg/day)			uric acid – clearance (ml/min)		
	basal	day 1.	day 2.	basal	day 1.	day 2.
controls (n = 9)						
x̄ ± MDM	594 ± 48	849 ± 151	673 ± 79	7.15 ± 1.68	10.07 ± 2.35	7.9 ± 1.32
signific.		s. ≦ 0.5%	s. ≦ 5.0%		s. ≦ 2.5%	n. s.
mixed ca. ox. (n = 11)						
x̄ ± MDM	728 ± 215	838 ± 138	841 ± 172	11.82 ± 3.39	13.20 ± 2.65	12.7 ± 2.44
signific.		n. s.	n. s.		n. s.	n. s.
pure ca. ox. (n = 17)						
x̄ ± MDM	529 ± 86	704 ± 180	643 ± 123	7.42 ± 2.24	9.47 ± 2.25	8.4 ± 1.48
signific.		s. ≦ 0.5%	s. ≦ 0.5%		s. ≦ 2.5%	n. s.
signific. mixed-pure ca. oxalate	s. ≦ 5%	s. ≦ 5.0%	s. ≦ 5.0%	s. ≦ 0.5%	s. ≦ 0.5%	s. ≦ 0.1%

MDM = mean deviation from the mean

In Table 3 the mean values of uric acid clearance can also be seen. From these values it is easier to recognize the inversely proportional connection between the serum and the urinary uric acid. On the first day in the control group there is a significant increase of uric acid clearance, followed by an almost normal level on the second day. In the mixed stone group the increase on both days is not significant; the significances of the patients with pure calcium oxalate stones are almost the same as those of the control group, but the temporal changes of the mean values are not greatly significant.

Besides the uric acid creatinine quotient, the uric acid GFR quotient was calculeted, to prove a greater significance of these two values (Table 4). The data shown in this table give no more information than the previous tables. During the test period the significances of the changing mean values within the different evaluations were similar in all groups.

The graph of the mean values of the urinary uric acid clearly shows the rapid increase of the uric acid excretion in the control group, followed by an equally fast decrease (Fig. 1). On the other hand, the increase of the mixed stone formers is much smaller and of no significance, remaining almost unchanged on the second day. There is also a clear increase in the pure calcium oxalate stones, but a smaller decrease on the second day.

The graph of the mean values of the uric acid clearance clearly shows the fast increase on the first day and the equally large decrease on the scond day for the control group

Table 4: Urinary uric acid/creatinine quotients and uric acid/GFR quotients after purine load

	urinary uric acid/creatinine (mg/g)			uric acid/GFR (mg/ml)		
	basal	day 1.	day 2.	basal	day 1.	day 2.
controls (n = 9)						
x̄ ± MDM	391 ± 83	492 ± 70	460 ± 79	5.20 ± 0.43	7.23 ± 1.05	6.23 ± 0.66
signific.		s. ≦ 5%	n. s.		s. ≦0.1%	≦ 0.5%
mixed ca. ox. (n = 11)						
x̄ ± MDM	459 ± 41	556 ± 94	538 ± 64	5.61 ± 1.20	7.71 ± 0.86	7.09 ± 0.95
signific.		s. ≦ 2.5%	s. ≦ 2.5%		s. ≦ 0.5%	s. ≦ 1%
pure ca. ox. (n = 17)						
x̄ ± MDM	433 ± 74	533 ± 106	519 ± 100	5.32 ± 1.20	7.19 ± 1.21	6.54 ± 0.79
signific.		s. ≦ 2.5%	s. ≦ 5.0%		s. ≦ 0.1%	s. ≦ 0.5%
signific. mixed-pure ca. oxalate	n. s.	n. s.	n. s.	n. s.	n. s.	n. s.

MDM = mean deviation from the mean

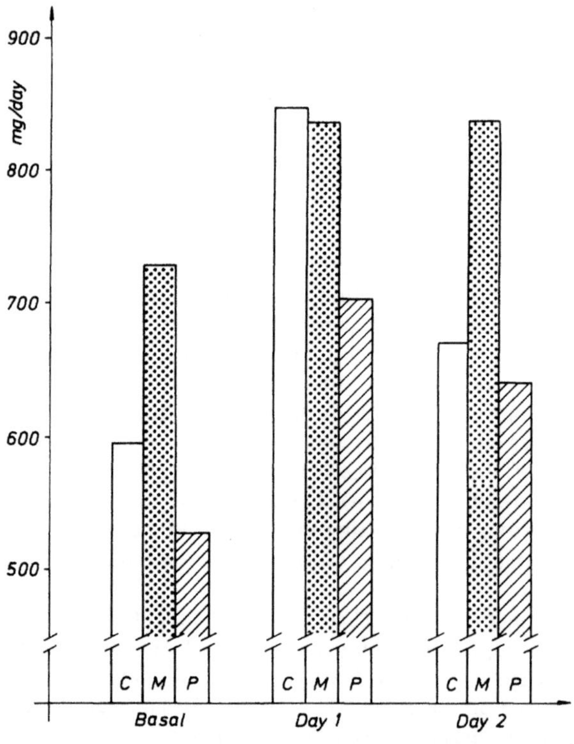

Fig. 1: Purine load: Urinary uric acid. C = controls, M = mixed Calcium oxalate, P = pure Calcium oxalate stones.

(Fig. 2). The mixed stone group shows a reduced increase on both days after purine load with constant clearance values, while in the group with pure calcium oxalate stones the changes of the values are almost the same as in the controls, but less significantly so.

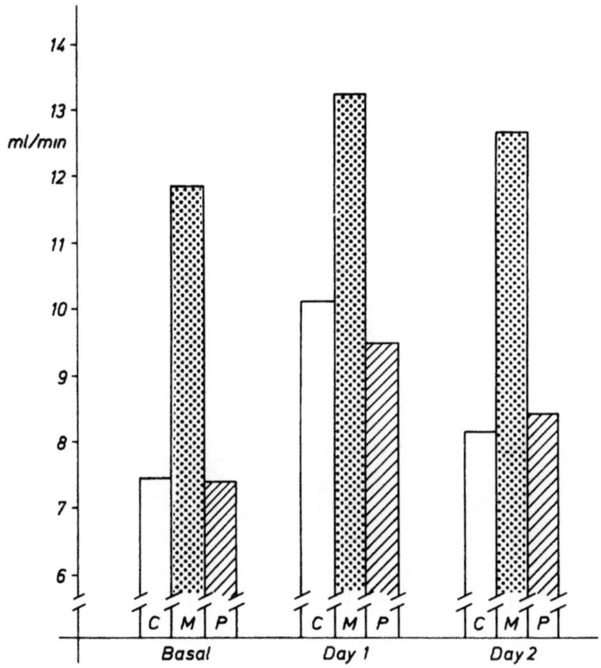

Fig. 2: Purine load. Uric acid clearance. C = controls, M = mixed Calcium oxalate, P = pure Calcium oxalate stones.

Discussion

Our evaluation of 28 urinary stone patients and 9 healthy controls proved that the serum uric acid in patients with calcium oxalate calculi compared with a control group within the first 24 hours after purine load is significantly higher than the vase value. On the other hand there is a highly significant increase of uric acid excretion in the control group and a non significant increase of uric acid excretion in the mixed stone group. Our results are partially contradictory to the evaluation of Bach and Schneeberger, who found a significant increase of uric acid concentration in serum and urine both in stone formers and healthy controls.

In our opinion the uric acid clearance is at present the best way of recognizing delayed uric acid elimination. The fluctuation of clearance values during the complete test period lead to this conclusion. Probably a better point of separation is to be found between normal and delayed uric acid excretion with variable dosage of the purine load and with a prolongation of the examination period.

Authors' address:

Dr. med. Bernhard Lux
Urologische Klinik des Allgemeinen Krankenhauses
Untere Sandstraße 32
8600 Bamberg
Germany

Prof. Dr. med. Jess Braun
Institut für Laboratoriumsmedizin des Allgemeinen Krankenhauses
Untere Sandstraße 32
8600 Bamberg
Germany

Fortschritte der Urol. und Nephrol. **16**, 81–87 (1981)
Steinkopff Verlag Darmstadt

Latent hyperuricemia and hyperuricosuria–a risk factor for stone formation–diagnosis with a purine-loading test

A. Hesse[1], W. Schneeberger[2], D. Bach[1], W. Dewes[3], and W. Vahlensieck[1]

1 Urologische Univ. Klinik Bonn
2 Rehabilitationskrankenhaus Bornheim-Merten
3 Physiologisch-Chemisches Institut der Univ. Bonn
West Germany

Increased uric acid in serum as a result of animal protein overconsumption and alcohol abuse is frequent nowadays. Concentrations above 6,5 mg uric acid/100 ml serum can lead to the deposition of uric acid or its salts in tissues, which in turn can lead to gout. Up to 40% of the patients suffering from gout also have uric acid nephrolithiasis. Without showing the symptoms of gout, however, uric acid stones as well as urate stones can form when the solubility product is exceeded either because of extreme uricosuria and/or because of an unfavorable urinary pH. About 20% of all urinary stones are totally or partially composed of uric acid or urate.

In the past uric acid has been recognized as significant for the genesis of Ca oxalate stones. The main mechanism discussed is a blockade of acidic mucopolysaccharides, which are considered to inhibit Ca oxalate precipitation (Robertson). The discovery of uric acid microliths (Berg) or sodium urate (Bellanato) in Ca oxalate stones has not been uncommon.

A latent hyperuricemia and slight hyperuricosuria can favor Ca oxalate stone formation. Therfore, it is of great importance for the evaluation of the pathogenesis and therapy to recognize the possible participation of uric acid in Ca oxalate stone disease.

When comparing serum uric acid in 57 Ca oxalate stone formers and 25 controls on unrestricted diet we found on average higher values in the patients. This is also evident when subdividing the groups into male and female (Tab. 1).

Table 1: Comparison of serum uric acid in Ca oxalate stone formers and healthy controls in relation to sex.

URIC ACID IN SERUM

Ca ox. stone formers mg/ 100 ml				healthy controls mg / 100 ml			
n		$\bar{x}$ ± SD		n		$\bar{x}$ ± SD	
17	♀	4.42 ± 1,39	5 - 6 n = 2 (11.8%) > 6 n = 1 (5.9%)	12	♀	3.88 ± 1.02	5 - 6 n = 1 (8,3%) > 6 n = 0
40	♂	5.89 ± 1,10	6 - 7 n = 12 (30.0%) > 7 n = 3 (7.5%)	13	♂	5.44 ± 0.60	6 - 7 n = 1 (7,7%) > 7 n = 0
57	♀+ ♂	5.45 ± 1,36	[1] path. n = 4 (7.0%) [2] latent n = 14 (24.6%)	25	♀+ ♂	4.69 ± 1.14	path. n = 0 latent n = 2 (8,0%)

[1] pathological value ≙ ♀ > 6, ♂ > 7
[2] latent hyperuricemia ≙ ♀ 5 - 6, ♂ 6 - 7

Table 2: Urinary uric acid excretion and concentration in Ca oxalate stone formers and healthy controls on individual diet.

URIC ACID IN 24-HOUR URINE ON INDIVIDUAL DIET			
Ca ox stone formers n = 24		healthy controls n = 25	
mmol/l	mmol/ die	mmol/l	mmol/die
2.5 ± 1.4	3.2 ± 1.5	2.6 ± 1.2	3.6 ± 1.3

Looking then at the urinary uric acid in 24-hour urine, no differences between the Ca oxalate stone patients and controls could be seen (Tab. 2).

In our special program for the diagnosis of urinary stones the influence of the individual diet is eliminated. The patients receive a so-called standard diet for 10 days, which is a balanced diet following the official nutrient recommendations. The liquid supply is restricted to either 1 400 ml or 2 400 ml per day.

Figures 1 and 2 show excretion and concentration of urinary uric acid in the standard diet with a daily liquid supply of 1 400 ml in 67 stone formers and 16 controls and 2 400 ml in 24 stone formers and 9 controls respectively. Again, no difference could be found in the urinary uric acid between stone formers and controls. From these figures we can see that on the standard diet a so-called "steady state" in the urinary components is reached on the 5th day, which we explain by the elimination of individual dietary habits. By increasing the daily liquid supply from 1 400 ml to 2 400 ml the urine is diluted (which means less concentrated); however, this effect is only significant in the controls. In stone formers the higher liquid supply leads to an increase in uric acid excretion.

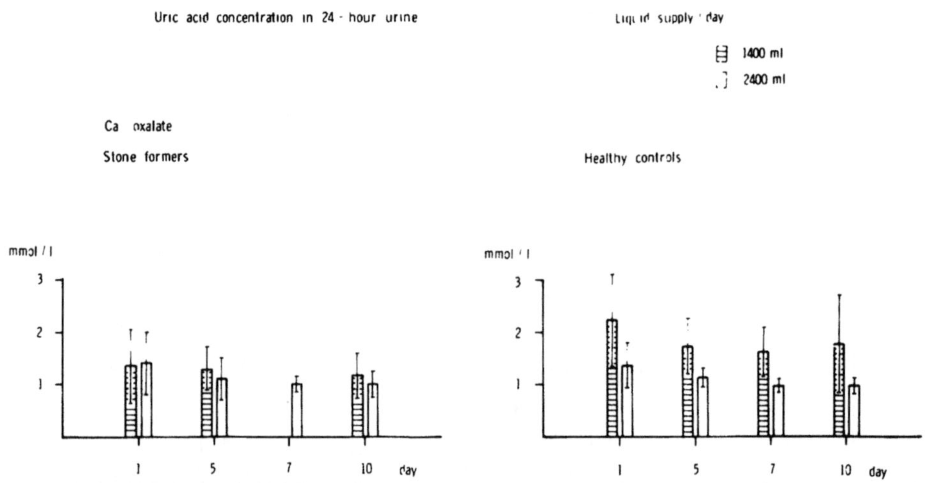

Fig. 1: Concentration of uric acid in 24-hour urine in Ca oxalate stone formers and healthy controls on a standard diet with different liquid supply.

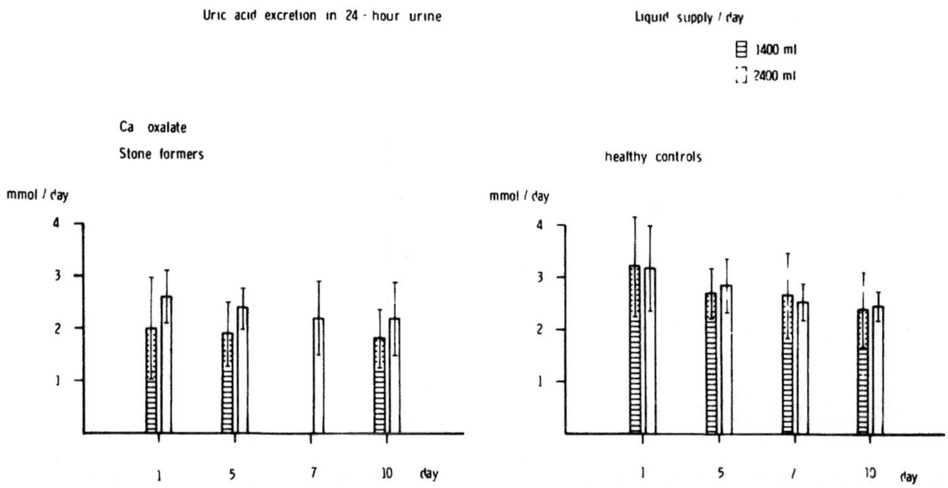

Fig. 2: Excretion of uric acid in 24-hour urine in Ca oxalate stone formers and healthy controls on a standard diet with different liquid supply.

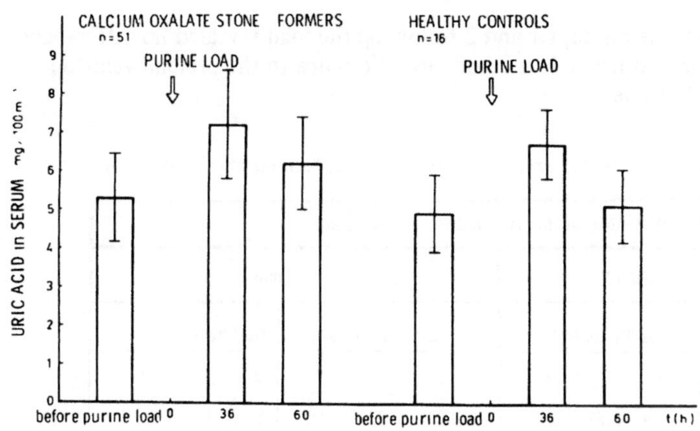

Fig. 3: Uric acid in serum after the purine loading test [Fa. Dr. E. Fresenius KG, Oberursel/Taunus (Germany)].

In recent years investigations have been carried out by our group with 2 g of a guanine/adenine mixture. Following this oral load the serum uric acid of Ca oxalate stone formers showed a significant increase, which remained for several days. In healthy controls the serum uric acid had returned to basic preload level on the second day after the load (Fig. 3).

Elimination of uric acid seems to be delayed in stone formers. Therefore, a purine load by the intake of purine-rich food might cause a hyperuricosuria for a longer period of time.

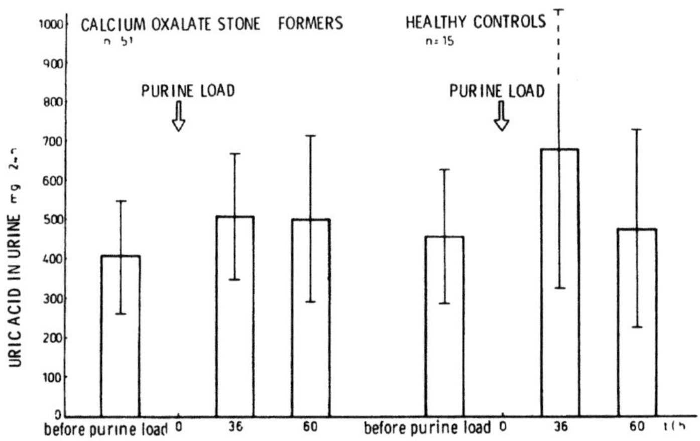

Fig. 4: Uric acid excretion in 24-hour urine following the purine loading test [Fa. Dr. E. Fresenius KG, Oberursel/Taunus (Germany)].

In Fig. 4 this is demonstrated under the conditions of the purine loading test. In the case of purine-rich food in combination with alcohol abuse a cumulative effect must even be expected.

Creatinine in serum and urine on days 1 and 2 following the load revealed no differences between stone formers and controls. Nor could any difference to the preload value be found, which is on day 0 (Table 3).

Table 3: Creatinine in serum and 24-hour urine in Ca oxalate stone formers and healthy controls.

CREATININ IN SERUM AND URINE FOLLOWING PURINE LOAD												
	SERUM (mg/ 100 ml)						URINE (mmol / die)					
	Ca ox. stone formers			healthy controls			Ca ox. stone formers			healthy controls		
Day	0	1	2	0	1	2	0	1	2	0	1	2
	0,98	1,04	0,89	0,89	0,87	0,89	14,1	12,8	11,3	14,4	12,3	11,7
n	12	12	5	9	9	7	18	18	18	11	11	11

Maxima in concentration and excretion of stone-forming substances in the circadian rhythm might resemble risk situations for stone formation. Therefore, patients and healthy controls collected the urine in a 3-hour postload specimen. We investigated all constituents that may play an important role in stone formation in these specimens.

In the excretion of uric acid a different course can be seen for stone formers and controls als demonstrated in Figure 5a and b for days 1 and 2 following the load.

The sinosoidal course of the circadian pH value is not influenced by the purine load (Fig. 6). The concentration of uric acid measured in each specimen never exceeds the value of

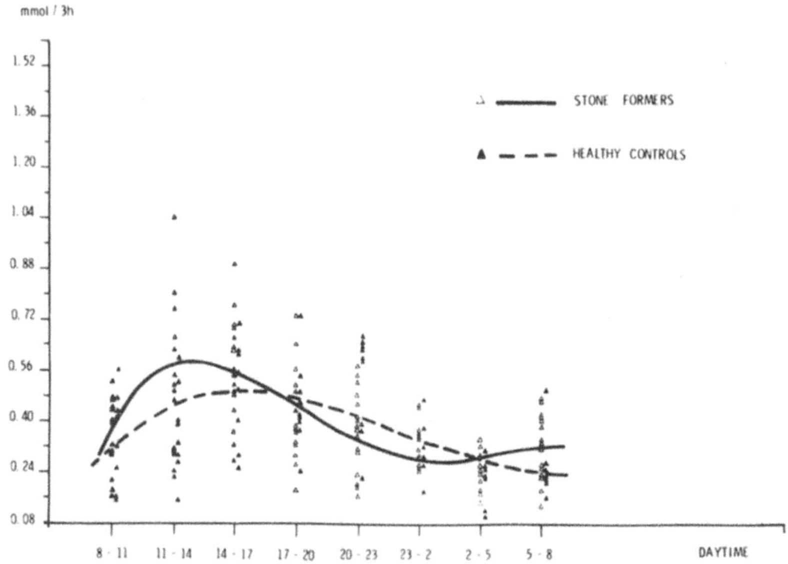

a

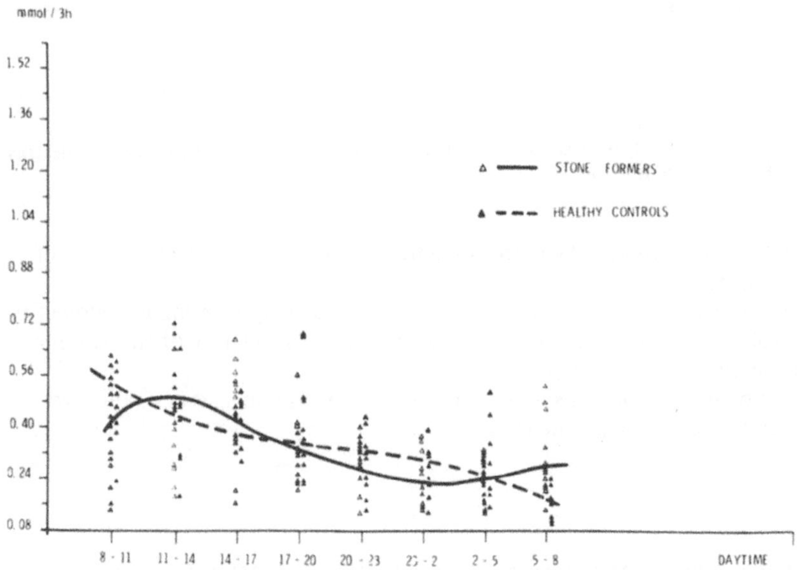

b

Fig. 5a and b: Circadian rhythm of uric acid excretion in Ca oxalate stone formers and healthy controls on day 1 (a) and day 2 (b) after the purine load.

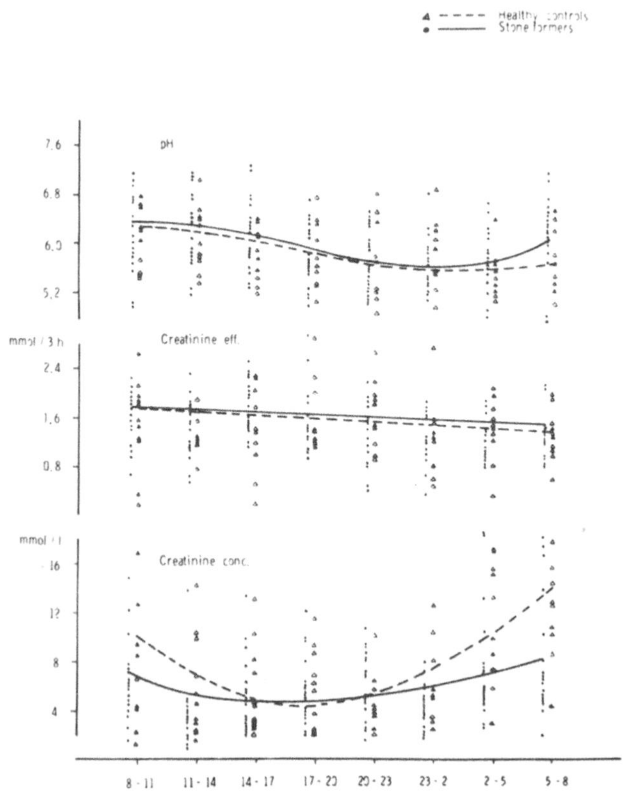

Fig. 6: Circadian rhythm of pH value and urinary creatinine in Ca oxalate stone formers and healthy controls on day 1 after the purine load.

4.5 mmol/liter. When looking at the corresponding pH value there is never a danger of uric acid crystallization.
No difference can be observed in the circadian rhythm of urinary creatinine in stone formers and controls at the time of the purine load and there is no change of this rhythm compared with preload conditions (Fig. 6).
Other urinary constituents such as sodium, potassium, calcium, magnesium, and citric acid are not influenced by the purine load.

Summary:

1. Serum uric acid is higher on average in Ca oxalate stone formers than in healthy controls.
2. There is no difference in the uric acid excretion of Ca oxalate stone formers on unrestricted and on standardized diet.

3. Following an oral purine load serum uric acid is significantly elevated in stone patients for several days. In healthly controls uric acid returns to preload values on the second day after the load.
4. Parallel to the increased uric acid in serum the urinary uric acid excretion remains elevated for several days in stone formers.
5. With the purine loading test latent hyperuricemia and hyperuricosuria can be diagnosed in stone formers, thus supporting effective prophylactical measurements.
6. The application of 2 g of a guanine/adenine mixture (1:1) could not reveal any side effects, and no changes in other constituents of serum and urine besides that of uric could be observed.

References

Berg, W., Schütt, S., Schneider, H.-J.: Polarisationsmikroskopische Untersuchungen zur Struktur und Genese von Harnsteinen: Jenaer Rundschau **23,** 188–192 (1978).

Bellanato, J., Cifuentes Delatte, L., Hidalgo, A., Santos, M.: Application of infrared spectroscopy to the study of renal stones. In: Urinary Calculi. Eds. Cifuentes Delatte, L., Rapado, A., Hodgkinson, A., Karger, S., Basel 1973, pp. 237–246.

Robertson, W.G., Knowles, F., Peacock, M., Urinary acid mucopolysaccharides inhibitors of calcium oxalate crystallization. In: Urolithiasis Research. Eds. Fleisch, H., Robertson, W.G., Smith, L.H., Vahlensieck, W., Plenum Press – New York and London 1976, pp. 331–334.

Author's address:

Dr. *A. Hesse*
Urologische Universitätsklinik Bonn
5300 Bonn 1 Venusberg
Germany

Fortschritte der Urol. und Nephrol. 16, 88–90 (1981)
Steinkopff Verlag Darmstadt

Laboratory Analysis of the Results of Treatment of Uric Acid Stones. "Zyloric U"—a New Insight (?)

K. Jarrar and W. Guttmann

Urologische Universitätsklinik, Gießen, West Germany

The effectiveness of allopurinol in the treatment of hyperuricemia and as a preventative against uric acid stone conditions has been clearly established. We do not think it necessary to go into the problem of the functioning of the xanthinoxydase inhibition since we assume that the comprehensive work of De Vries and Sperling (1976) is familiar to everyone.
Numerous clinical studies have demonstrated a significant lowering of abnormally high uric acid level in the serum and 24-hour urine of hyperuricemia and uric acid stone patients after treatment with allopurinol.
However gastrointestinal side effects have necessitated the development of a new form of Zyloric, Zyloric U, which is available in granular form. Bach und Schneeberger have shown in a crossover study that there is no difference between Zyloric 300 and Zyloric U as far as their clinical effectiveness is concerned. On the other hand, treatment with Zyloric U noticeably reduced the gastrointestinal side effects.

Our test methods

20 patients (15 male, 5 female) with normal uric acid function, a history of uric acid stones, and abnormally high serum and uric acid stones, and abnormally high serum and uric acid levels were treated over a period of 7 months with Zyloric U. Before the commencement of outpatient treatment the following readings were taken:
intravenous urogram, minor blood analysis, urine status, and uricult, serum concentration in 24-hour excretion of urine substances (creatinine, uric acid, urea, electrolytes [Na, K, Ca, Mg], and the excretion of the trace elements iron, copper, and zinc).
Electrolyte and trace element determinations in the urine were varried out by flame atom absorption spectroscopy. Only by this method and by using a long suction time of 6–8 ml is it possible to determine the very low copper concentrations. This allows calculation of mean values with low mean standard deviations (RSD) from numerous single values of the digital multimeter. An attenuation of at least 3 seconds is recommended, as copper concentrations in the urine are slightly above the sensitivity limit of flame spectroscopy. Under these technical conditions it is advantageous to use the flame rather than the graphite tube cuvette.
The treatment began with a daily dose of one 300 mg sachet of Zyloric U. The above-mentioned readings were repeated every 6 weeks.

Results

Possible side effects were evaluated along with the therapeutic effectiveness and the laboratory analysis. In the case of one patient it was necessary to terminate the treatment because of painful swellings in the joints and extremities. The patient had no history of gout. The statistical evaluation of the laboratory analysis was carried out in the Medical Statistical Institute of Gießen University (Fräulein Olfert, Director: Prof. Dudek). A double variation analysis was employed as the method of evaluation. The first checks showed a reduction of the uric acid readings from the initial pretreatment readings of 8.36 ± 0.61 to 5.76 ± 1.84 mg/100 ml. These readings remained relatively constant, so that at the end of the treatment the average serum uric acid reading was below 6.3 mg/100 ml. The average uric acid excretion was approximately 320 mg in the 24-hour urine. In the case of *zinc* the variation among test persons was so great that no definite conclusions could be drawn about changes during the test period. None of the other parameters showed any noticeable change during therapy, with the exception of copper. As Fig. 1 shows, the treatment with Zyloric U is followed by a noticeable rise in the copper level, followed by a significant fall in a later phase. The reason for this can be seen as a change in the metabolism, which, however, we have not as yet been able to interpret clinically. We consider, however, that proved change in copper level could be a very reliable indicator for objective control residual stone prophylaxes.

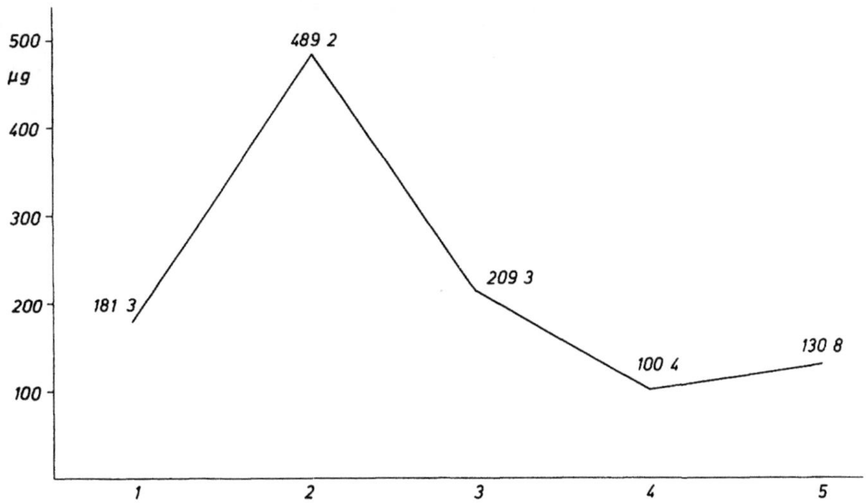

Fig. 1: Copper levels in 24-hour urine at 5 six-week intervals.

The copper level readings showed:
1. that the differences between test persons were determined by chance.
2. between measurements there were differences with a margin of error of less than 5%.

The final test urogram showed no negative effects. A cherry-sized, X-ray negative kidney stone of one female patient had been reduced to the size of a hazel nut during the 6-month period of treatment. The patient reported that a relatively high excretion of fine crystals in her urine had taken place, without colics. Another female patient reported much the same except that in her case multiple excretion of fine crystals had taken place, accompanied by dull pains.

Author's address:

Dr. *K. Jarrar*
FA für Chirurgie und Urologie
Dr. *W. Guttmann*
FA für Innere Krankheiten
Urologische Klinik der
Universität Gießen
Hinter der Ostanlage 5
6300 Gießen
Germany

Fortschritte der Urol. und Nephrol. **16**, 91–98 (1981)
Steinkopff Verlag Darmstadt

The Action of a Benzbromarone-Citrate Preparation on Lithogenous and Inhibitory Substances

D. Bach, A. Hesse, A. Strenge, and W. Vahlensieck

Urologische Universitätsklinik Bonn, West Germany

Uric acid bears a very close relation to urinary stones. Uric acid stones appear very often in patients with a high uric acid blood concentration and increased uric acid excretion in the urine. But an increase of uric acid in urine can also promote the formation of calcium oxalate stones because uric acid blocks the inhibitory activity of the acid mucopolysaccharides on the precipitation of calcium oxalate (6).

One object of prophylaxis of uric acid- and calcium oxalate stones must therefore be the permanent lowering of uric acid levels in blood and urine (1, 10, 11). The uricostatic-acting allopurinol is mainly used in such treatments with great success. Uricosuric substances, which also significantly decrease the serum uric acid, have until now met with much criticism from urologists in their use as a prophylactic agent (1, 4, 8, 9) because at the beginning of each uricosuric therapy the elimination of uric acid is greatly increased. If the solubility capacity for uric acid is exceeded, this leads to precipitation of uric acid crystals, even when the urinary pH is within the physiological limits. The increased risk of stone formation can be avoided by adequate urinary dilution and the raising of the urinary pH to 6.5–6.8.

When benzbromarone is combined with citrate there are two resulting guaranteed effects –normalization of the serum uric acid and improvement of their solubility in urine.

We examined the preparation Harolan®, an effervescent granulate which is composed of 50 mg benzbromarone and 2.4 g of a mixture of citric acid and citrate (Tab. 1).

Table 1: Composition of Harolan® granulates

Benzbromarone	50 mg
Citric acid	678 mg
Potassium citrate	1 189 mg
Sodium citrate	539 mg
Sodium hydrogen carbonate	462 mg

(Producer: Fa. Merz + Co., Frankfurt a. M., W. Germany)

We wanted to determine the following:

1. The extent of serum uric acid decrease,
2. The average level of the elimination of uric acid after the administration of Harolan,
3. The extremes of pathological concentration resulting from this process in the circadian rhythm,
4. Whether the citrate-induced raising of the urinary pH promotes the increase of solubility of uric acid, and
5. Should an influence on other lithogenous and inhibitory substances be observed?

Materials and Methods

1. Patients

A total of 36 patients with calcium oxalate stones were examined for ten days. The patients ranged in age from 33 to 74 years. We treated 21 patients (group I) with the benzbromarone-citrate combination (Harolan®). 15 patients (group II) remained without therapy and served as a control group.

2. Examination

All patients received a standard diet during the 10 days. This diet complied with the regulations of the German Association of Nutrition and eliminates the variabilities of nutritional supply which we established in the metabolic examination of our kidney stone patients who have suffered relapses (12).
The daily liquid intake was 2 400 ml. After attaining a "steady state" on the 5th day—that is, the elimination and concentration of lithogenous and inhibitory urinary substances displayed insignificant change—patients in group I received for 5 days an intake at 8 a. m. of one bag of Harolan (= 2.45 g).
Table 2 shows the parameters which were determined in serum and urine for both groups. We determined the initial values on the day before starting the therapy—that means the 5th day on standard diet or day 0 in the course of therapy with Harolan®.
After starting the therapy blood analysis took place daily in group I, in group II only once on the 4th day of treatment.

Table 2: Measured constituents in serum and urine

Serum	Urine
Uric acid	Urine volume
Creatinine	pH
Calcium	Uric acid
Magnesium	Citric acid
Phosphate	Creatine
	Sodium
	Potassium
	Magnesium
	Calcium
	Phosphate
	Sulfate
	Chloride

The examination of 24-h urine also took place daily in both groups with one difference: on the 4th day of treatment the urine was collected in 3-h portions and the circadian rhythm of the stone-related substances was then determined. The evaluation was followed by a statistical program developed in our Urolithiasis Research Department (3).

Results

1. Blood concentrations

After only two days, group I, which was treated with Harolan®, attained a significant decrease in uric acid (up to 50% of the initial values) and was recorded throughout the duration of the examination (Fig. 1). In comparison, the uric acid levels of the control group II remained the same. The serum values of Na, K, Ca, Mg, P, and creatinine remained within the normal range for both groups and revealed no differences over the entire period of examination.

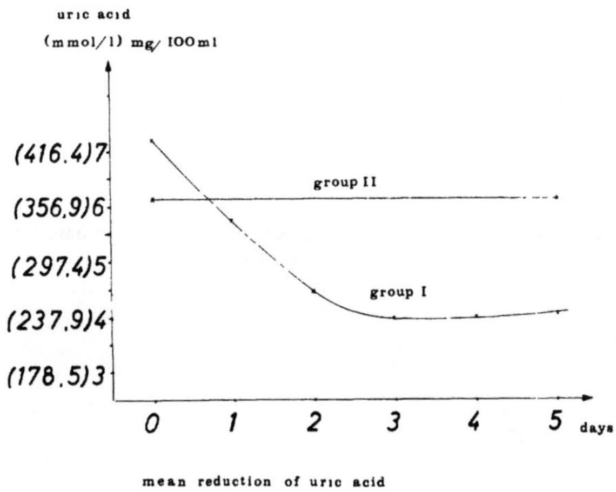

Fig. 1: Concentration of uric acid plotted against time.

2. Urinary concentration and excretion

2.1. 24-h urine

2.1.1. Uric acid

The uric acid concentration and elimination rose in group I on the 1st and 2nd day after the therapy began at mean values of 1.74 mmol/l and 4.42 mmol/24 h respectively (Fig. 2). However, the uric acid concentration never attained values which could have promoted the crystallization of uric acid (Fig. 3). In group II the concentration and elimination of uric acid remained unchanged throughout the examination.

2.1.2. Urinary pH

The average urinary pH in group I increased constantly from 6.0 to a stabilized value of 6.4 to 6.6 (Fig. 4). In the control group, the pH average remained at approximately the same level of 6.0 for the duration of the examination.

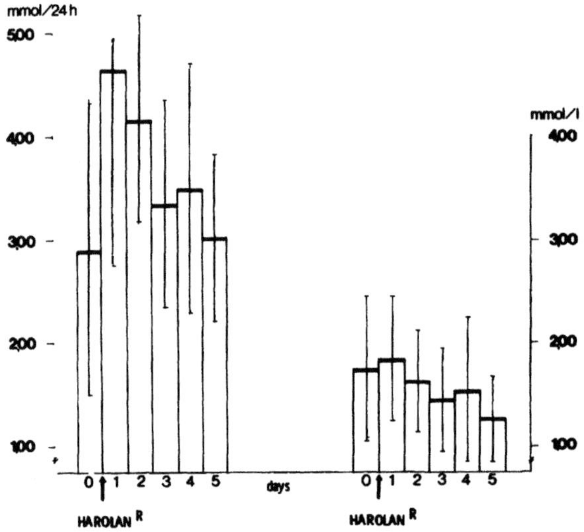

Fig. 2: Excretion and concentration of uric acid in 24-h urine after application of a benzbromarone-citrate mixture (Harolan®) in 21 calcium oxalate stone formers on standard diet.

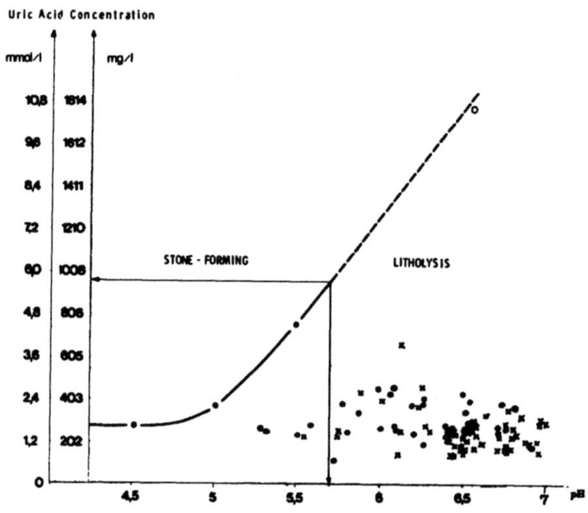

Fig. 3: Solubility of uric acid in synthetic urine (Berenyi 1972) and uric acid values of 21 calcium oxalate stone formers • on 1st and 2nd day with Harolan®. x on 3rd, 4th, and 5th day with Harolan®.

2.1.3. Citric acid

The kidneys displayed an increased elimination of citric acid through the raising of the pH (Fig. 5). This finding coincides with results of examinations performed by Butz und

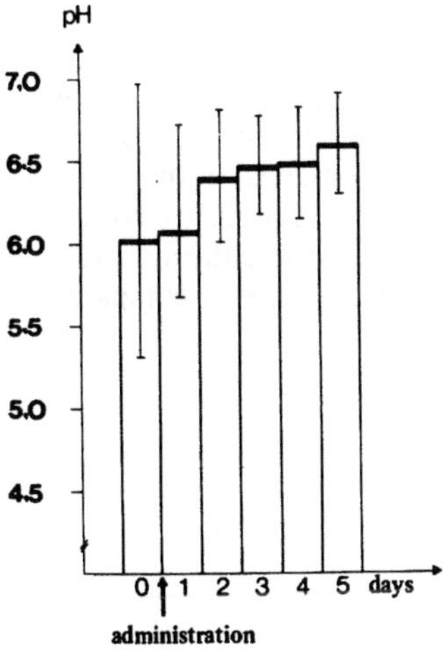

Fig. 4: pH-value of 24-h urine under standard diet and application of a benzbromarone-citrate mixture.

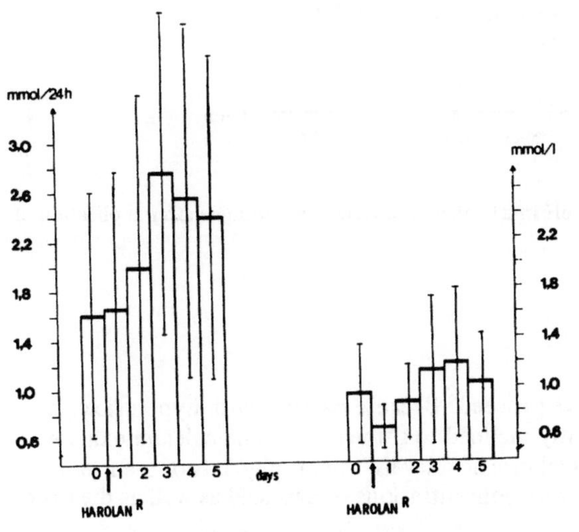

Fig. 5: Excretion and concentration of citric acid in 24-h urine after application of a benzbromarone-citrate mixture (Harolan®) in 21 calcium oxalate stone formers on standard diet.

Dulce (2), which indicated that an increase in excretion of citric acid is displayed with the application of alkaline salts of citric acid. However, because of the wide standard deviations in our results, the increase in concentration and excretion of citric acid is not significant.

Other Parameters

During the entire examination, the excretion and concentration of Na, K, Cl, Mg, P, S, and creatinine showed no significant differences.

2.2 Circadian Rhythms

The wave-like circadian graph of the excretion and concentration of uric acid exhibited by patients in group I on the 4th day of Harolan therapy indicated no elevation of the uric acid concentration. Only an elevation of excretion has been observed in the first three hours after Harolan® application. In comparison, there was a very clear increase in the urinary pH (Fig. 6). In group II the circadian rhythm of uric acid concentration and excretion showed a similar trend. We found no significant differences in comparison to group I.

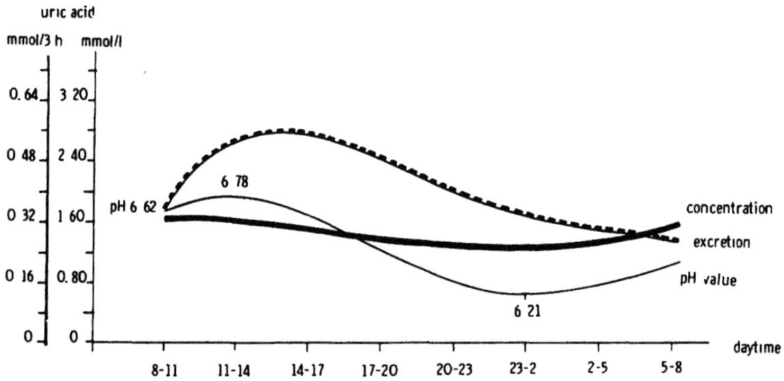

Fig. 6: Circadian rhythm of uric acid and pH in 21 calcium oxalate stone formers after application of Harolan®.

Discussion

Along which lines of reasoning shall we proceed? Because patients with hyperuricemia and hyperuricosuria are more frequently inclined to get uric acid- and calcium oxalate kidney stones than patients with normal uric acid levels, the prophylaxis of recurrent stones can result from a decrease in serum concentrations of uric acid as well as the excretion of uric acid in the urine.

As a rule, allopurinol fulfills this purpose. However, it is not unusual to find that there are situations where allopurinol cannot be utilized because it can lead on the one hand to symptoms of intolerance. On the other hand, sometimes the desired decrease of the serum uric acid cannot be obtained despite increased doses.

There is the possibility of utilizing an uricosuricum in combination with a citrate mixture. As we have seen, an uricosuricum can produce initial hyperuricosuria – but does not induce an increased risk of formation of uric acid- and calcium oxalate crystals. At no time in the therapy did the uric acid content in urine reach a level which could have encouraged crystallization.

In addition, the risk of uric acid stone formation is lessened through the increase of urine dilution and the maintenance of urinary pH by the citrate components.

The benzbromarone-citrate composition of Harolan® complies with this. We could confirm the former documented decrease of serum uric acid from our studies. The urinary pH remains between 6.4 to 6.6 from the 3rd day.

An increase of uric acid excretion and concentration only became apparent on the first two days after the beginning of the therapy. The initial value was again attained after the 3rd day. At no time was the level of urinary uric acid such as would encourage uric acid crystallization.

The circadian rhythm shows that the increased uric acid concentration was compensated for by the simultaneous increase of the pH. The citrate excretion and concentration was raised.

According to our results, one can use the benzbromarone-citrate mixture in patients with uric acid- or calcium oxalate stones when an increased serum uric acid value is used as an indication (5).

Patients with healthy kidneys receiving longterm treatment with benzbromarone are not expected to display bromide accumulation. 50 mg of benzbromarone contains 18.85 mg bromide. Even if the entire amount is reabsorbed and set free from its organic ties, this would result in a bromide pool of 336.5 mg in the steady state. Proceeding from a volume distribution where the plasma volume alone is approximately 2 500 ml, one would reckon with a maximal bromide concentration of between 13 and 14 mg/100 ml serum. Side effects normally only appear with serum concentrations of at least 150 to 200 mg/100 ml.

Summary

The benzbromarone-citrate mixture Harolan® was examined in 21 calcium oxalate stone formers for its value as a prophylactic agent in the treatment of relapses of uric acid- and calcium oxalate stones. The examinations were administered in conjunction with a standard diet in an effort to eliminate the variabilities of excretion of lithogenous and inhibitory substances through individual eating habits.

The use of Harolan® can induce a significant decrease of serum uric acid by the simultaneous raising of the urinary pH through better solubility for the increase of uric acid excretion in the first two days. In 24-h-urine and in the circadian rhythm the uric acid solubility graph was never exceeded during the examination. No side effects were observed.

References

1. Bach, D., W. Vahlensieck: Therapie und Rezidivprophylaxe des Harnsteinleidens. DMW **105:** 783 (1980).
2. Butz, M., H.J. Dulce: Enhancement of urinary citrate in oxalate stone formers by intake of alkaline salts in: L.H. Smith, W.G. Robertson, B. Finlayson (Eds.): Urolithiasis, New York–London, Plenum Press 1981.
3. Dewes, W., D. Bach, M. Rohde, H. Kurth: Beschreibung eines Verfahrens zur Bestimmung von Kurvenverläufen mittels Polynome anhand von Beispielen aus der Harnsteinforschung. EDV in Med. Biol. **11:** 59 (1980).
4. May, P., B. Lux: Gichtbehandlung und -prophylaxe mit Urikosurika. Dtsch. Ärztebl. **74:** 1593 (1977a).
5. Mertz, D.P.: Intraindividueller Wirkungsvergleich von 300 mg Allopurinol mit 100 mg Benzbromaron. Therapiewoche **28:** 6080 (1978).

6. Robertson, W.G., F. Knowles, M. Peacock: Urinary Acid Mucopolysaccharide Inhibitors of Calcium Oxalate Crystallisation. Urolithiasis Research (Eds.: H. Fleisch, W.G. Robertson, L.H. Smith, W. Vahlensieck) New York–London, Plenum Press, p. 331, 1976.
7. Rugendorff, E.W., S. Barsom, M. Schulte: Harnsäuresenkung und Harnsäuresteinprophylaxe unter verschiedenen Benzbromaronzubereitungen. Therapiewoche **30:** 6597 (1980).
8. Samberger, N., J. Braun, B. Lux, P. May: Harnsäuresteinbildung und Uratverstopfung der ableitenden Harnwege durch Urikosurika. Aktuelle Urologie **10:** 21 (1979).
9. Vahlensieck, W.: Methodik der peroralen Chemolitholyse und Dauer der Prophylaxe bei Harnsäuresteinen. Med. Welt **21,** 1559 (1970).
10. Vahlensieck, W.: Konservative Therapie der Urolithiasis. Med. Welt **29:** 2 (1978).
11. Vahlensieck, W. (Hrsg.): Urolithiasis 5: Der Harnsäure-, Zystin-, Xanthinstein. Berlin–Heidelberg–New York, Springer 1980.
12. Vahlensieck, W., D. Bach, A. Hesse, W. Schneeberger: Metabolic Investigations in 407 Recurrent Stone Formers and Healthy Controls on Condition of Individual as well as Standard Diet in L.H. Smith, W.G. Robertson, B. Finlayson (Eds.): Urolithiasis, New York–London, Plenum Press 1981.

Author's address:

Dr. *Dietmar Bach*
Urologische Universitätsklinik Bonn
Sigmund-Freud-Str. 25
5300 Bonn Venusberg
Germany

Fortschritte der Urol. und Nephrol. 16, 99–105 (1981)
Steinkopff Verlag Darmstadt

Pathogenesis and Incidence of Calcium-containing and Pure Uric Acid Stones in Patients with Hyperuricemia and Hyperurocosuria

P. May, B. Lux, and J. Braun

Urologische Klinik und Insitut für Laboratoriumsmedizin des Allgemeinen Krankenhauses Bamberg, Akademisches Lehrkrankenhaus der Universität Erlangen, West Germany

There are several factors which can be involved in the formation of pure uric acid stones: The first of these is the steady acidity of the urine. In addition to the absolute concentration of uric acid, the pH of the urine has a critical influence on the formation of uric acid stones.

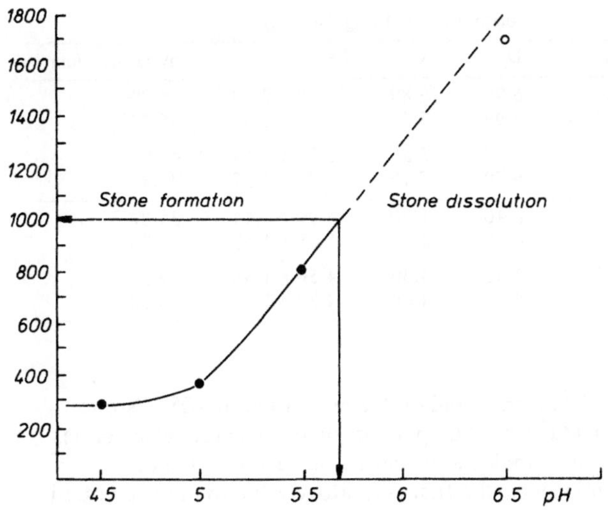

Fig. 1: Solubility of uric acid dependent on pH value.

Fig. 1 shows how much the solubility of uric acid depends upon the pH value. For the so-called idiopathic uric-acid-stone-diathesis without hyperuricemia and hyperuricosuria, the only characteristic clinical indication is the low pH of between 4.8 and 5.5 compared to the normal values of healthy persons of 5.7 to 6.3 – this is in cases when there is no stone formation. The relative "continuity of the acidity of the urine" – which according to investigations by Atsmon, Gutman, and Sperling is caused by a reduced elimination of ammonia – is also found in most gout patients. In 1978 Yü and Gutman determined in 47% of their gout patients a constant low pH of the urine of between 4.8 and 5.0.

Table 1: Frequency of hyperuricemia and hyperuricosuria in patients with pure uric acid calculi

author	year	hyperuricemia	hyperuricosuria
Dulce	1962	–	75%
Zöllner	1968	33%	33%
Bressel	1971	20%	–
Sramek	1973	46%	52%
Kollwitz	1974	33%	–

The frequency rate of patients with idiopathic uric acid stones without hyperuricemia and hyperuricosuria varies. Table 1 shows the widely differing percentages of various authors.

Table 2: Frequency of hyperuricemia in uric acid calculi

			serum uric acid (mg/100 ml)			
year	calculi	n	D	x	x ± s	hyperuricemia
1977	♂ primary	54	6.99	6.89	7.09 ± 2.39	46.3%
	recurrent	48	6.99	7.22	7.72 ± 2.59	56.3%
	♀ primary	31	5.33	5.56	5.97 ± 2.14	41.9%
	recurrent	30	6.79	7.19	7.05 ± 2.37	73.3%
1980	♂ primary	80	6.40	5.90	5.90 ± 1.44	35.0%
	recurrent	73	6.00	5.50	5 68 ± 1.50	37.0%
	♀ primary	35	4.30	4.30	4.50 ± 1.38	29.0%
	recurrent	26	4.60	4.60	4.87 ± 1.30	38.5%

Table 2 shows our own findings: They are based on the evaluation of 1055 "stone-patients" during 1977 and on an additional 565 patients in 1980. Serum electrolytes and urine analyses on 24-hour urine samples were carried out on all of them.
Paying no attention to the control values, the first laboratory value found was enterd into our statistics. This was done to find evidence of how often pathological serum and urine values were present in just one checkup. On the other hand, all analyses which showed a serum creatinine value above 1.4 mg/100 ml or a creatinine-clearance below 80 ml/min. were neglected, to exclude the possibility a renal insufficiency being the cause for the pathological laboratory values.
To gain a more complete impression on the distribution of the data of the analyses, additional statistical values – besides the mean value – were determined, as can be seen from the tables.
The two groups of patients examined – one in 1977 and the other in 1980 – differ from each other insofar as the older group of patients consisted mainly of inpatients

from the urological clinic of the university of Homburg/Saar while the 1980 group consisted of 50% inpatients and 50% outpatients treated at the urological clinic in Bamberg. Laboratory tests were performed in all cases by Dr. Braun. The frequency of the percentage of patients with hyperuricemia among those who had developed uric acid stones varied between 29 and 73%. The percentage of recidive stone patients is generally higher.

Table 3: Frequency of hyperuricosuria in uric acid calculi

			urinary uric acid (mg/day)			
year	calculi	n	D	x	x ± s	hyperuricosuria
1977	primary	48	483	525	572 ± 327	22.9%
	recurrent	50	663	750	774 ± 326	46.0%
1980	primary	73	531.0	577	622 ± 209	28.8%
	recurrent	74	551.3	539	599 ± 170	27.0%

From Table 3 it can be seen that one group shows a clear-cut difference in the percentage frequency of increased uric acid elimination into the urine between primary and recidive stone patients, while the 1980 group shows that the frequency is generally a little below 30%.

Increased uric acid elimination is not only caused by gout and hereditary hyperuricemia but also partly occurs following the application of certain pharmaceuticals. Urologists observe that – when there is a longer drugs – there is a development of uric acid stones. More often, however, there appears to be a blocking of the ureters by urates which may have extended into the state of a lingering ureamia.

Table 4: Frequency of urinary stasis in patients with uric acid lithiasis

total	529	
pure uric acid calculi	161	(30.4%)
Frequency of urinary stasis in uric acid stones with and without treatment with uricosuria:		
total	161	
with urinary stasis	133	(82.6%)
bilateral	15	(9 %)
serum creatinine over 2 mg%	56	(34.8%)
urinary stasis in uric acid stones treated with uricosurica	33	(20.5%)

Out of 529 inpatients with nephrolithiasis, in 30.4% these stones consisted of pure uric acid (Table 4). In 133 of 161 patients with uric acid stones, which means in almost 83%, the concrement had led to a congestion of the descending urinary tract; this occurred on both sides in 15 cases. As can also be seen from Table 4, in more than 20% of the cases a treatment with a uricosuricum – generally Benzbromaron – had been started.

With the clinical findings of frequent congestion by urates and the formation of uric acid stones in the descending urinary tract after a longer Benzbromaron application in mind, the question was posed, whether a hyperuricosuria caused by Benzbromaron might be responsible for these findings.

Table 5: Increase of uric acid elimination in 24 h urine samples after Benzbromaron treatment (100 mg daily)

	pre	day 1.	day 2.	day 3.	day 4./5.	day 6./7.	week 2.	week 3./4.	week > 4.
n =	20	10	12	11	13	18	13	12	6
uric acid (mg/day)									
x	500	1050	800	863	950	900	1038	750	950
x	566	1113	863	913	918	909	989	797	1052
± s	138	252	167	276	165	258	188	164	230
uric acid increase %									
x		70.0	50.0	67.5	41.7	50.0	70.0	35.0	113.0
x		101.0	61.0	65.2	63.0	53.3	73.3	38.9	112.0
± s		56.9	42.6	45.7	53.7	33.4	28.1	16.8	77.2

Table 5 shows the results of a trial over 4 weeks and longer on uric acid elimination determined from 24-hour samples collected from 20 healthy persons, who – along with a normal intake – were given daily in the morning 100 mg Benzbromaron tablets. It can be seen that – along with a significant decrease of serum uric acid – there is a rapid increase of uric acid in the urine. As soon as the day following the first Benzbromaron application, the uric acid value had risen up to 1100 mg/day, and up to 900 mg/day on the following days. This is equivalent to 60% more than the initial value.

Table 6: Increase of uric acid clearance after Benzbromaron treatment (100 mg daily)

	pre	day 1.	day 2.	day 3.	day 4./5.	day 6./7.	week 2.	week 3./4.	week > 4.
n =	20	10	12	11	13	18	13	12	6
uric acid clearance (ml/min)									
x	5.6	20	19	21	22.8	18	16	26.7	25
x	6.0	21.1	19.5	23.2	23.2	21.0	19.9	23.1	22.0
± s	1.8	6.5	4.2	9.1	8.3	9.2	11.0	10.4	9.0
uric acid clearance increase %									
x		275	217	275	269	266	250	275	288
x		270	237	290	295	261	265	276	348
± s		129	97	149	150	125	182	175	191

Table 6 demonstrates the significant increase of the uric acid clearance values, determined in the same 20 healthy test persons, who – as before – were given 100 mg Benz-

bromaron daily. The highest of these values was that of a 22-year-old man. He showed a normal value to start with and then after 3 weeks his uric acid content rose up to 3200 mg in 24-hours and after another 3 weeks (6 weeks Benzbromaron application altogether), he had a uric acid value of 1800 mg 24-hours.
Without wanting to discuss the working mechanism of Benzbromaron more closely, which, according to Zöllner, is only based upon the uricosuric effect, it should be mentioned that from the urological point of view a longer lasting application of Benzbromaron can lead to urate obstruction and uric acid stone formation in the descending renal tract, if there is no satisfactory diuresis and alkalization of the urine.
According to Zöllner up to 40% of all gout patients aquire nephrolithiasis. There are – as found Gutman an Yü – not just uric acid stones involved, but in 12% of the gout patients calcium stones were also discovered; these were mainly stones of calcium oxalate.
Table 7 shows the frequency of the percentage of hyperuricemia in patients with calcium oxalate stones. A percentage varying from 25 to almost 36% in different groups of test persons can be seen. The percentages of hyperuricemia in patients with mixed calcium oxalate stones are a little lower (Table 8).

Table 7: Frequency of hyperuricemia in calcium oxalate calculi

			serum uric acid (mg/100 ml)			
year	calculi	n	D	x	x ± s	hyperuricemia
1977	♂ primary	56	5.38	5.92	6.28 ± 1.85	35.7%
	recurrent	84	6.25	6.28	6.48 ± 1.95	31.0%
	♀ primary	108	4.78	5.04	5.08 ± 1.46	28.7%
	recurrent	75	4.82	5.03	5.20 ± 1.58	33.3%
1980	♂ primary	48	4.75	5.45	5.40 ± 1.03	25.0%
	recurrent	41	5.50	5.50	5.42 ± 1.30	26.82%
	♀ primary	23	4.90	4.40	4.46 ± 0.65	26.08%
	recurrent	28	3.60	3.75	4.01 ± 1.10	32.14%

Table 8: Frequency of hyperuricemia in mixed calcium oxalate calculi

			serum uric acid (mg/100 ml)			
year	calculi	n	D	x	x ± s	hyperuricemia
1980	♂ primary	40	5.60	5.45	5.37 ± 1.26	22.5%
	recurrent	45	5.10	5.30	5.50 ± 1.11	28.9%
	♀ primary	33	4.70	4.00	4.18 ± 1.17	18.2%
	recurrent	29	5.00	3.80	4.08 ± 0.99	24.1%

Hyperuricosuria has been found to be a decisive factor in the formation not only of uric acid stones, but also, as we know today, of calcium-containing concrements, these being primarily calcium oxalate stones (Table 9). The frequency of a hyperuricosuria in patients with calcium oxalate stones was found to range from 23 to 47%.

Table 9: Frequency of hyperuricosuria in calcium oxalate calculi

year	calculi		n	urinary uric acid (mg/day) D	x	x ± s	hyperuricosuria
1977	oxalate	total	36	650	700	708 ± 243	47.2%
	mixed	primary	64	492	533	594 ± 287	20.3%
	oxalate	recurrent	74	509	559	588 ± 203	29.7%
1980	oxalate	primary	71	688	632	635 ± 172	32.3%
		recurrent	69	683	600	620 ± 225	23.2%
	mixed	primary	73	531	577	622 ± 209	29.0%
	oxalate	recurrent	74	551	539	599 ± 170	27.0%

Table 10: Percentage frequency of increased uric acid in serum and urine

year	type of stone		hyperuricemia *and* hyperuricosuria
1977	oxalate	total	13.9%
	mixed oxalate	total	10.3%
	uric acid	total	25.0%
1980	oxalate	primary	9.9%
		recurrent	10.1%
	mixed oxalate	primary	4.1%
		recurrent	7.0%
	uric acid	primary	4.3%
		recurrent	8.0%

While it is easy to understand that there is crystallization and uric acid stone formation in a urine saturated with uric acid, there are various explanations for the induced formation of calcium-containing stones due to increased uric acid elimination.

On account of clinical observations which demonstrate that a considerable percentage of patients with calcium oxalate stones show an increased uric acid elimination, the authors Kallistratos (1970) and even more so Coe (1975) were able to present evidence by in vitro investigations that after adding crystallized sodium urate a precipitation of calcium oxalate crystals can be brought about from a metastable solution.

On the other hand there is the opinion of Robertson, who emphasizes the influence of the uric acid concentration of the urine on the formation of calcium-containing concrements ments due to the process of crystallization. He assumes that increased uric acid concentration stops the blocking activity for crystallization of calcium oxalate, which derives from the acid mucopolysaccharides.

Whatever the theory, in cases of patients with uric acid as well as calcium oxalate stones who suffer, in addition, from hyperuricemia or hyperuricosuria it is vital to apply a Zyloric treatment to lower the increased serum and especially also the urine uric acid concentration.

Summary and Conclusion

Serum and urine analyses of 2 large groups of test persons show, that hyperuricemia and hyperuricosuria rather frequently cause – or are part of the cause of – the formation of uric acid stones, although a steady urine acidity must be considered to be the most important factor for the crystallization of uric acid. Last but not least iatrogenic hyperuricosuria must be mentioned, which includes the formation of uric acid stones and the blocking of the ureters by urates following a longer lasting therapy with uricosuric drugs, especially when care is not taken for a satisfactory diuresis and alkalization of the urine. The correlation between uric acid metabolism and calcium oxalate stone formation is indicated by the high incidence of hyperuricemia and hyperuricosuria found in patients with calcium oxalate stones.

References

Alken, C.E., P. May, J. Braun: Harnsteinleiden – Thieme – Stuttgart (1979).

Atsmon, A., A. De Vries, M. Frank: Uric acid lithiasis. Amsterdam–London–New York: Elsevier (1963).

Berenyi, M.: Ein Nierensteinmodell. In: Die Harnsäure und Urate. 2. Jenaer Harnsteinsymposium. Hrsg. v. E. Hienzsch und H.S. Schneider. Wiss. Beitr. d. Friedrich-Schiller-Universität Jena, S. 56 (1972).

Braun, J., P. May: Harnsäureuntersuchungen im Serum und Urin. Ein Vergleich bei Harnsäure- und Oxalat-Steinbildnern. Fortschr. Urol. Nephrol. **7:** 115 (1975).

Braun, J., P. May: Klinisch-chemische Analysen bei Harnsteinpatienten. Fortschr. Urol. Nephrol. **9:** 254 (1977).

Bressel, M.: Klinik und Therapie der Harnsäure-Nephrolithiasis. In: Fettsucht –Gicht, hrsg. von W. Boecker. Thieme – Stuttgart 182 (1971).

Coe, F.L., R.L. Lawton, R.B. Goldstein, V. Tembe: Sodium urate accelerates precipitation of calcium oxalate in vitro. Proc. soc. exper. Biol. **149:** 926 (1975).

Dulce, H.J.: Über die Harnsteinpathogenese. Internist **3:** 884 (1962).

Gröbner, W., N. Zöllner: Uricosurica, aus Gicht – Handbuch der Inn. Med. 7, 3, 491 (1976) hrsg. v. N. Zöllner und W. Gröbner, Springer-Verlag, Berlin–Heidelberg–New York.

Gutman, A.B., T.F. Yu: Uric and metabolism in normal man and primary gout. N. Engl. J. Med. **273:** 313 (1965).

Kallistratos, G., A. Timmermann, O. Fenner: Zum Einfluß des Aussalzeffektes auf die Bildung von Calciumoxalatkristallen im menschlichen Harn. Naturwissenschaften **57:** 198 (1970).

Kollwitz, A.A., H. Kracht, R. Brauer, E. Löhe: Klinische- und Laborbefunde bei 470 Patienten mit Kalziumsteinen der oberen Harnwege. Urol. Int. **24:** 318 (1969).

May, P., J. Braun, W. Menke: Behandlungsergebnisse beim Harnsäuresteinleiden. In: Nieren- und Hochdruckkrankheiten **3:** 126 (1974).

Mertz, D.D.: Uratnephrolithiasis. Ursache oder Folge. Fortschr. Med. **94:** 1160 (1976).

Samberger, N., J. Braun, B. Lux, P. May: Harnsäuresteinbildung und Uratverstopfung der ableitenden Harnwege durch Uricosurica. Akt. Urol. **10:** 21 (1979).

Sramek, F.: Die Anwendung von Zyloric beim Uratsteinleiden. In: 3. Jenaer Harnstein-Symposium, Wiss. Beitr. der Friedrich-Schiller-Universität Jena 1973 (S. 167).

Yü, F.: Uric and Nephrolithiasis. In: Uric acid. Handbook of Experimental Pharmakology. Vol. 51, Kelley, W.N., Weiner, J.M. (eds.) Berlin–Heidelberg–New York, Springer (1978), p. 397.

Zöllner, N.: Die interne Behandlung des Harnsäuresteinleidens. Urologe **7:** 46 (1968).

Zöllner, N., W. Gröbner: Häufigkeit der Nephrolithiasis bei Gicht, aus Gicht-Handbuch der Inn. Med. 7, 3, 371 (1976), hrsg. von N. Zollner und W. Gröbner, Springer-Verlag, Berlin–Heidelberg–New York.

Author's address:

Prof. Dr. Peter May
Urologische Klinik
des Allgemeinen Krankenhauses
Untere Sandstraße 32
8600 Bamberg
Germany

Fortschritte der Urol. und Nephrol. **16**, 106–109 (1981)
Steinkopff Verlag Darmstadt

Clinical Characteristics of the Calcium Stone Disease in Hyperuricosuria

U. Backman, B. G. Danielson, B. Fellström, G. Johansson, S. Ljunghall and B. Wikström

Department of Internal Medicine, University Hospital, Uppsala, Sweden

Introduction

Two possible roles of urate in calcium stone formation have been suggested. One is stone formation through epitaxy as the structure of urate and calcium oxalate crystals are rather similar. Another suggested mechanism is that urate acts as an anti-inhibitor of precipitation and growth of calcium oxalate crystals.

Several authors have considered a high urinary urate as a risk factor for calcium stone formation (1, 2). The frequency of hyperuricosuria among calcium stone formers has also been reported to be rather high by some authors (1, 3).

However, for a critical evaluation, a proper selection of controls is mandatory. In the present study the urinary urate was determined in recurrent stone formers and in an age- and sex-matched control group. An evaluation of the clinical picture was made in those cases who were considered to have a high excretion of urate.

As we have earlier shown a high incidence, 20%, of defective tubular acidification (RTA) in recurrent stone formers (4), consideration was also given to this defect in the present study during evaluation of the clinical picture.

Material and method

At our out-patient stone clinic, 467 consecutive recurrent stone formers, 350 men and 117 women, were examined with regard to urate metabolism. The urate excretion in stone formers was compared with the excretion in 89 healthy subjects recruited from a health survey.

Hyperuricosuria was defined as urate excretion exceeding the mean plus one standard deviation found in healthy subjects, which corresponds to 4.0 and 4.5 mmol/24 hours for females and males respectively. So defined, hyperuricosuria was found in 57 subjects. These 57 patients were compared with an age- and sex-matched group of stone formers who had normal excretion of urate. All patients were investigated ambulatorily on their ordinary diet. Urate was measured with an enzymatic spectrophotometric method. Lithium carbonate ($LiCO_3$) was used as a preservative for urinary collections. Renal acidification capacity was investigated with a short-term ammonium chloride load (5).

Results

The urinary excretion of urate was the same in stone formers as in stone-free control persons. In females the excretion was lower than in males (Table 1). In the females the excretion decreased with advancing age.

Table 1: Urinary excretion of urate in control persons and recurrent calcium stone formers

	Controls	*Stone formers*
Males		
n	51	350
Age	41.5 ± 18.2	45.7 ± 13.1
Urinary urate	3.5 ± 1.1	3.3 ± 1.0
Females		
n	37	117
Age	49.6 ± 19.8	40.2 ± 14.0
Urinary urate	2.9 ± 0.9	3.0 ± 0.9

The frequency of hyperuricosuria, according to our definition, and renal acidification defects (RTA) are presented in Table 2. Ten patients who had both hyperuricosuria and RTA had the incomplete form of the defect. Eight had the proximal form and the other 2 the distal form. In the normouricosuric group 7 had the proximal type and 3 the distal type, all of the incomplete form. The duration of the stone disease was the same in both groups. Hyperuricosuric patients had a high operation rate. But when consideration was taken of acidification defects, only hyperuricosuric patients with RTA exhibited the higher operation rate (Fig. 1).

Table 2: The frequency of hyperuricosuria and renal acidification defects (RTA) in recurrent calcium stone formers

Some metabolic findings in stone formers

	Males	*Females*
Hyperuricosuria (♀ > 4.0 mmol/24h ♂ > 4.5 mmol/24h)	46 (13%)	11 (9%)
RTA	43 (12%)	36 (31%)
Hyperuricosuria + RTA	6 (2%)	4 (3%)

Discussion

In the present study the definition of hyperuricosuria was set at a moderately increased excretion of urate, namely, the mean of the values found in healthy subjects plus one standard deviation. The reason for this definition was that only a few patients, about 3–4%, had an excretion over the 95% tolerance limit. In order to have a larger number of patients for evaluation of the clinical picture, a wider limit was chosen.

The possible role of urate as a risk factor for calcium stone formation has been much discussed (1, 2, 6). If a high urinary urate was a general risk factor, the excretion of urate should be higher in stone formers than in controls. Our results could not confirm this, as there was no difference between stone formers and control persons with regard to the excretion of urate. Other investigators have reached diverging results (1, 2, 3). The reason

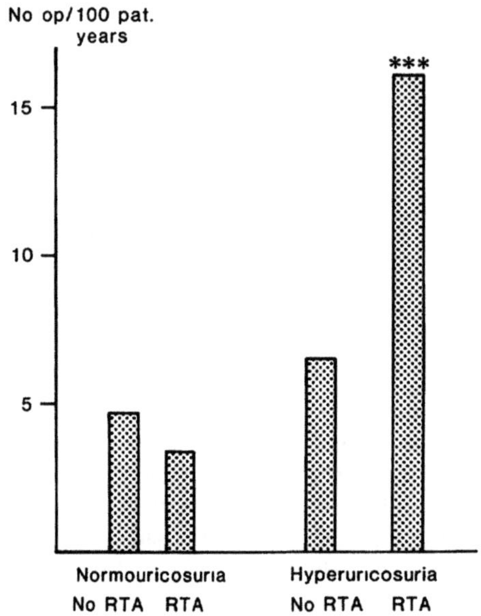

Fig. 1: The operation rate (stone operations/100 patient-years) in stone formers with normouricosuria and hyperuricosuria. In both groups ten patients had RTA.

for this difference is not quite clear, but dietary differences may explain the deviation between various parts of the world.

Although a high urinary urate might not be a general risk factor, hyperuricosuric individuals could have particular clinical features. For a proper evaluation of the clinical characteristics it is also important to have an age- and sex-matched control group as the urate excretion varies with these factors. Our hyperuricosuric stone formers had an increased operation rate compared to matched normouricosuric patients. This finding has been confirmed by other investigators (7). However, metabolic factors could also have influenced the stone formation in our group. We have earlier found a rather high frequency of renal acidification defects (20%) in recurrent stone formers (4) and these cases also had a higher operation rate than other stone formers. When consideration was taken of RTA in this study the high operation rate was found only in those cases who had both hyperuricosuria and RTA. Thus, it seems possible that RTA is a more important factor for calcium stone formation than a high urate excretion.

In conclusion, urate excretion in this study was the same in recurrent stone formers and healthy control persons. Hyperuricosuric stone formers had the same clinical picture as normouricosuric patients. Only hyperuricosuric patients who also had RTA had a higher operation rate. Thus, the opinion that urate should be regarded as a common risk factor for calcium stone formation is not supported by this study.

References

1. Robertson, W.G., Peacock, M., Heyburn, P.J., Marshall, D.H., Clark, P.B.: Risk factors in calcium stone disease of the urinary tract. Brit. J. Urol. **50:** 449–454 (1978).

2. Coe, F.L., Kavalach, A.G.: Hypercalciuria and hyperuricosuria in patients with calcium nephrolithiasis. New Engl. J. Med. **291**: 1344–1350 (1974).
3. Smith, M.J.V., Hunt, L.D., Cling, J.S., Boyce, W.H.: Uricemia and urolithiasis. J. Urol. **101**: 637–642 (1969).
4. Backman, U., Danielson, B.G., Johansson, G., Ljunghall, S., Wikström, B.: Incidence and clinical importance of renal tubular defects in recurrent renal stone formers. Nephron. **25**: 96–101 (1980).
5. Backman, U., Danielson, B.G., Sohtell, M.: A short duration renal acidification test. Scand. J. Urol. Nephrol. **35 (suppl)**: 33–48 (1976).
6. Hodgkinson, A.: Uric acid disorders in patients with calcium stones. Br. J. Urol. **48**: 1–5 (1976).
7. Coe, F.L.: Treated and untreated recurrent calcium nephrolithiasis in patients with idiopathic hypercalciuria, hyperuricosuria or no metabolic disorders. Ann. Int. Med. **87**: 404–410 (1977).

Author's address:

Dr. *U. Backman*
Dept. of Internal Medicine
University Hospital
750 14 Uppsala
Sweden

Fortschritte der Urol. und Nephrol. **16**, 110–113 (1981)
Steinkopff Verlag Darmstadt

β_2-Microglobulin Excretion in Patients with Uric Acid Stones

K.-H. Bichler, S. Korn, I. Lämmert, and A. Haußmann

Department of Urology, University of Tübingen, West Germany

For the pathogenesis of urine acid lithiasis, tubular defects must be considered. These defects are possibly connected with changed urine acidity and enzymatic defects. Our own previous examinations of patients with uric acid stones showed a significant decrease of uromucoid excretion, a fact, which we would like to interpret as an alteration in the tubular region. In this connection the question arises whether patients with uric acid lithiasis have proteinuria resulting from a tubular insufficiency. Tubular defects can lead to typical proteinuria, especially the excretion of β_2-microglobulin (Wibell). Its determination in the urine is suitable for the diagnosis of the tubular proteinuria.
The following are some facts about β_2-microglobulin: It is a low molecular weight protein with a M.W. of about 12 000 and is found in all body fluids. β_2-microglobulin is freely filtered at the glomerulus and is reabsorbed to more than 99.9% and catabolzed in the proximal tubuli. In patients with tubular disorders with proteinuria the GFR is normal or slightly reduced and the β_2-microglobulin level in the serum is normal or slightly elevated and β_2-microglobulin excretion in the urine is elevated. With chronic renal insufficiency GFR is severely impaired, and the β_2-microglobulin level is elevated in the serum and the urine. We have measured the β_2-microglobulin excretion in the urine and serum in order to determine these changes. For the measurement of β_2-microglobulin excretion a radioimmunoassay of Pharmacia (Phadebas® β_2 micro test, Pharmacia Uppsala) was used. In addition we controlled the uromucoid excretion (by Electroimmunodiffusion according to Bichler), the GAG excretion (according to Blumenkrantz and Asboe-Hansen), and the citrate excretion (according to MacArdle and Knappwost). Urine acid excretion and urine pH were also determined.
We examined altogether 17 patients: 9 men and 8 women. The patients were aged between 20 and 75 years. Two stones were found in the urine, 15 in the renal pelvis. We selected a patient group with uric acid percentage of 90–100% in the analysis of their urinary calculi.

Results

The values of β_2-microglobulin excretion in the urine were 30–370 μg/24 hours. The level in the serum was 0.8 to 2.4 μg/ml. The results of 5 of 17 patients, that is 29,4%, showed an increased β_2-microglobulin excretion in the urine ranging between 938 and 10 000 μg/24 hours. In the serum we found an increased β_2-microglobulin level in 11 of 17 patients, that is 64.7%. The values lay between 2.97 and 9.6 μg/ml. 4 of 17 patients showed uric acid excretion ranging between 600 and 979 mg/24 hours. A typical urinary acidity of about 5.4 we found in 14 of 17 patients, that is 82.3%.
The uromucoid excretion in 11 of 17 patients was (64.7%) decreased. The range was 6.0 to 29.5 mg/24 hours. The GAG excretion in 8 of 17 patients with urinary acid stones

was 1.0 to 4.5 mg/24 hours. So here it is decreased. The urinary citrate in patients with uric acid stones was in 70.5% (12 of 17) decreased. The range was 58 to 325 mg/24 hours.

There is a good correlation between the concentration of β_2-microglobulin and creatinine in the serum (fig 1). In 64.7% of the patients we found an increased β_2-microglobulin level in the serum, possibly in connection with the tubular alteration. The β_2-microglobulin level in the serum is a good semiquantitive parameter of the glomular filtrate. The reduced glomular rate of filtration leads to a measureable rise of β_2-microglobulin concentration. The reduction of uromucoid and citrate excretion in 60 to 70.5% of the patients we would like to interpret as a tubular alteration.

Comparing β_2-microglobulin excretion in patients with calcium oxalate, uric acid, and struvite stones it can be seen that the patients with struvite stones have the highest values (fig 2). This can be taken as a result from a pyelonephritic tubular alteration.

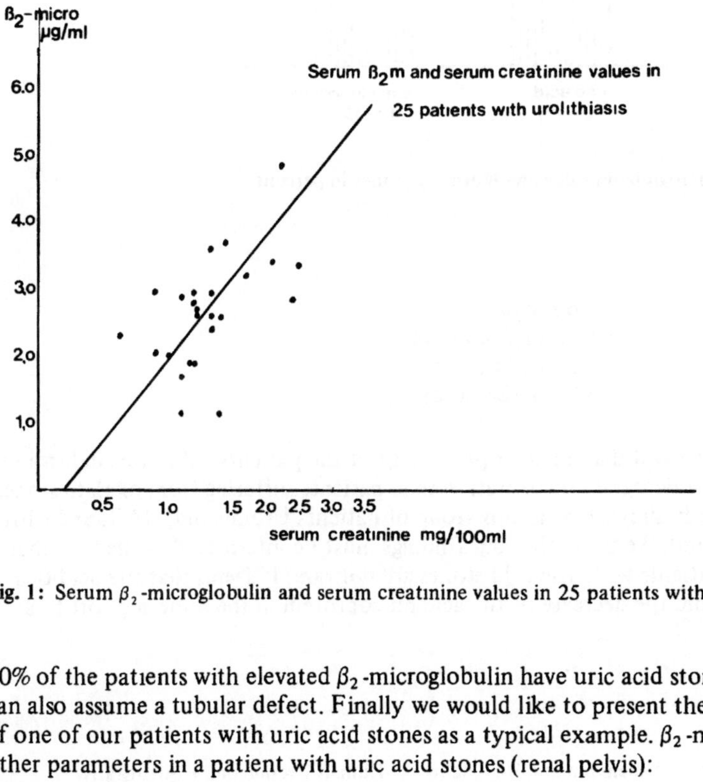

Fig. 1: Serum β_2-microglobulin and serum creatinine values in 25 patients with urolithiasis.

30% of the patients with elevated β_2-microglobulin have uric acid stones. In this case we can also assume a tubular defect. Finally we would like to present the laboratory values of one of our patients with uric acid stones as a typical example. β_2-microglobulin and other parameters in a patient with uric acid stones (renal pelvis):

M. K. 70 years

Stone analysis:	95% uric acid	
Urine pH	5.3	
β_2-microglobulin	urine	938 µg/24 hours
	serum	3.70 µg/ml

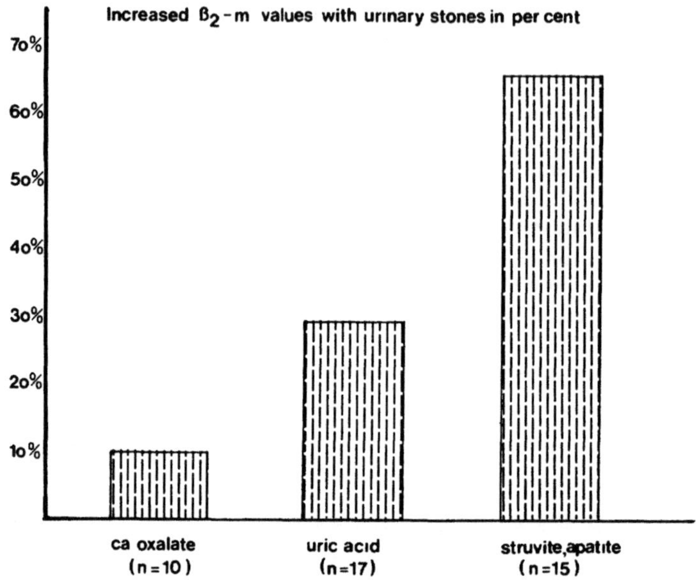

Fig. 2: Increased β_2-microglobulin values with urinary stones in percent.

Creatinine	1.60 mg%
Uromucoid	13.0 mg/24 hours
GAG	7.5 mg/24 hours
Citrate	325 mg/24 hours

Summerizing it can be said that a higher percentage of the patients with uric acid stones have an increased β_2-microglobulin excretion than patients suffering from oxalate stones. Furthermore our study shows that in this group of patients Uromucoid, GAG, and Citrate excretion are decreased. We think that our findings must be interpreted in the way that tubular defects in patients with uric acid stones are not rare. It seems that the acidification, reabsorption, and the decrease of the acid mucoprotein in the urine support this hypothesis.

References

K.-H. Bichler, H. Haupt, G. Uhlemann and H.G. Schwick: Human Uromucoid. I Quantitative immunoassay. Urol. Ress. **1:** 50 (1973).

H. Blumenkrantz und G. Asboe-Hansen: A new method for the quantitative determination of uronic acids. Anal. Biochem. **54:** 484 (1973).

B. MacArdle: A modified method for the micro-determination of citrate Biochem. J. **60:** 647 (1955).

A. Knappwost, S. Gerlach: Zur Methodik der Zitratbestimmung im Harn. In: Pathogenese und Klinik der Harnsteine. V.G. Gasser and W. Vahlensieck ed. Steinkoff, Darmstadt, 1977.

L. Wibell: Studies of β_2-microglobulin in human serum, ure and amniotic fluid. Doctoral Thesis at Uppsala University (1974).

Author's address:

Prof. Dr. *K.H. Bichler*
Lehrstuhl und Abteilung für Urologie
der Universität Tübingen
7400 Tübingen
Germany

GPSR Compliance

The European Union's (EU) General Product Safety Regulation (GPSR) is a set of rules that requires consumer products to be safe and our obligations to ensure this.

If you have any concerns about our products, you can contact us on ProductSafety@springernature.com

In case Publisher is established outside the EU, the EU authorized representative is:

Springer Nature Customer Service Center GmbH
Europaplatz 3
69115 Heidelberg, Germany

Batch number: 10577969

Printed by Printforce, the Netherlands